NATUR. TREATMENTS
For The World's
220
Most   Common
Ailments

PLUS

A Complete Guide
To
Vitamins - Minerals
Herbs
Amino Acids
+
Tissue Salts

Dear Reader

This highly acclaimed international best selling guide has been completely revised and updated for the nineties, providing the general public with the latest breakthroughs in vitamin and herb science. It is the most comprehensive, concise and straight forward natural health guide on the market today. Simplified, allowing you to skim through and find what you want and need to know when you're at your busiest, or digest at your leisure. Using the quick scan index, clearly designed charts on vitamins, minerals, herbs, amino acids and tissue salts, you get more information in less reading time. That's precisely why busy people like you around the world rely on the Vitamin & Herb Guide.

Global Health keeps you in touch with the proper natural treatments and remedies for the world's most common ailments. Also included, quick reference R.D.A. charts. Effects and side effects of the common vitamins, minerals, and herbs and in which foods they can be found. We are united in cause, to help you restore health, prevent premature aging, and prolong life. This guide will expand your awareness of treating yourself as naturally as possible, and discover a comfortable relationship with the latest natural alternatives for your busy lifestyle.

Global Health wishes to thank the following individuals for their time, energy, dedication and support in the preparation of the book.

Our sincere thanks to ...

Pearl Chapman	-	Research
Mark Ferguson	-	Research
Ann Brown	-	Research
Louise Kitura	-	Research
Gordon Ramsey	-	Research
Laura Rinas	-	Research
Betty Gervais	-	Research, Editing
Jim Patterson	-	Editing
Joan Davis	-	Typesetting
Margaret Lammerts	-	Cover Design, Artwork

David H. Nyholt
President, Global Health Ltd.

INDEX

220 OF THE WORLD'S MOST COMMON AILMENTS

World's ailments
(continued)

INDEX

A WORD ABOUT HERBS

SINGLE HERBS

A herb with medical properties used by Herbalists for the prevention and correction of disease. All herbs in this book are presented for the express purpose of making it easy for the layman to use.

HERBAL COMBINATIONS

Herbal combinations consist of two or more herbs selected and compounded to cover symptoms of specific diseases. A single herb often does not have all of the therapeutic qualities that are required.

220 OF THE WORLDS MOST COMMON AILMENTS

ACNE.....

HERBAL COMBINATION :AKN
PHYSIOLOGIC ACTION: Acne is nearly always the product of blood impurities. AKN helps cleanse toxins and mucus. Enhances overall good health and well-being, and helps eliminate skin blemishes and acne.
SINGLE HERBS: Burdock, Chaparral, Chlorophyll, Echinacea, Garlic, Gotu Kola, Red Clover, and Yellow Dock.
VITAMINS: A, B complex, B3, B6, C, E, and F.
MINERALS: Potassium and Sulfur.
ALSO: Primadophilus.
REFERENCES:
"Acne" — J. Howland
"Global Herb Manual" — Zeke Fortisevn

AIDS.....

(Acquired Immune Deficiency Syndrome)
SINGLE HERBS: Cayenne, Chinese Ginseng, Garlic, Milk Thistle, Pau d'Arco, Shiitake Mushroom, Sheep Sorrel, Suma, and Yucca.
VITAMINS: A, B6, B12 B complex (stress), and E.
MINERALS: High potency mulimineral formula, plus Copper, and Zinc.
ALSO: Canaid herbal drink, Acidophilus, Coenzyne Q10, Germanium, Gluconic from DaVinci Labs, Proteolytic Enzymes, Raw Thymus, and Multiglandulars.
REFERENCES:
"Complete Natural Health Encyclopedia" - David Nyholt

"Natural Treatments & Remedies"—Global Health

AIR SICKNESS.....
Refer to Motion Sickness Pg. 36

ALCOHOLISM.....

HERBAL COMBINATIONS:
(Thisilyn) (Milk Thistle) (PC) (Liveron) (AdrenAid).
PHYSIOLOGIC ACTION: The above herbal formulas support and rebuild the liver, pancreas, and adrenal glands. By supporting these systems, the taste for alcohol will eventually subside. The vitamin and mineral supplements strengthen the body's nutritional integrity to a state where the need for a "lift" will be eliminated.
SINGLE HERBS: Cayenne, Dandelion, Siberian Ginseng, Golden Seal, Licorice Root, Lobelia, Nettle, Skullcap, and Valerian.
VITAMINS: A, B complex, C, D, and E.
MINERALS: Brewers Yeast, Magnesium and Zinc.
ALSO: Glutamine, and Tryptophan. Avoid meat and all refined and processed foods, especially white sugar and white flour.
REFERENCES:
"Herbally Yours"—P. Royal
"How to get Well"—P. Airola

ALLERGIES.....

HERBAL COMBINATION:
(HAS: Original and Fast Acting Formulas) (AllergyCare)
PHYSIOLOGIC ACTION: HAS is an excellent formula which contains herbs that help relieve symptoms of hay fever, sinus congestion, and respiratory allergies. Helps drain nasal passages, relieve swollen membranes, eliminate mucus, and cleanse the body. The Fast Acting Formula

adds Pseudoephedra, a natural plant extract from the Ephedra plant. This substance quickly opens nasal passages allowing free breathing. While HAS Fast Acting is not for prolonged use, HAS Original can be taken for as long as needed.
Caution: Both formulas are not to be used during pregnancy.
Allergy Care: Maximum-strength natural allergy medicine that will not cause drowsiness. It contains 60mg of the active ingredient Pseudo ephedrine Hcl.
Caution: Not to be used during pregnancy, nor by small children.
SINGLE HERBS: Burdock Root, Cayenne, Chaparral, Elderberry, Eyebright, Lobelia, Golden Rod, Golden Seal, and Nettle.
VITAMINS: A, B complex, B3, B5, B6, B12, C, E, and F.
MINERALS: Calcium, Magnesium, and Manganese.
ALSO: Bee Pollen, Propolis, and Digestive Enzymes.
REFERENCES:
"Allergy"—W. Crook
"Every Woman's Book"—P. Airola

ALOPECIA .....
Refer to "Baldness" Page 11

ANEMIA .....
(Iron deficiency anemia)
SINGLE HERBS: Barley Grass, Beet Powder, Black Current, Chlorophyll, Chorella, Comfrey, Dandelion, Fenugreek, Kelp, and Yellowdock.
VITAMINS: A complete multivitamin and additional C.
MINERALS: Complete multi-mineral.
ALSO: Dessicated liver.

ANGINA .....
Refer to "Myocardial Infraction" Page 37

ARTERIOSCLEROSIS
HERBAL COMBINATION: (Garlicin HC)
PHYSIOLOGIC ACTION: A combination of herbs which supports the cardiovascular system. Helps to strengthen the heart, while building and cleansing the arteries and veins.
SPECIFICS: Recent animal studies suggest that vitamin C deficiency could be involved in the causation of arteriosclerosis. E.F.A.s (essential fatty acids) play a fundamental role in keeping cell membranes fluid and flexible.
SINGLE HERBS: Cayenne, Comfrey, Evening Primrose Oil, Fish Oil, Garlic, Golden Seal, and Rose Hips.
VITAMINS: B complex, C, E, Niacin, Inositol, and Choline.
MINERALS: Calcium and Magnesium.
ALSO: (E.F.A.s) — Fish oils and cold pressed vegetable oils.
REFERENCES:
Evening Primrose Oil - J. Graham
"Fats and Oils" - U. Erasmus

ARTHRITIS AND RHEUMATISM .....
HERBAL COMBINATION: (Rheum-Aid) or (Yucca -AR)
PHYSIOLOGIC ACTION: Relieves symptoms associated with bursitis, calcification, gout, rheumatoid arthritis, rheumatism, and osteoarthritis. Helps the body reduce or eliminate swelling and inflammation in the joints and connective tissue and helps to relieve stiffness and pain.
SINGLE HERBS: Alfalfa, Black Cohosh, Burdock, Chaparral, Devil's Claw, and Yucca.
VITAMINS: Niacin, B, C, D, E, F, and P.
MINERALS: All.

ALSO: Cod liver oil, green magma, aqua life, seatone, bromelain, papaya, cherry juice, pineapple, goats milk, and mung beans.
REFERENCES:
"There is a Cure for Arthritis"
"How to Get Well"— P. Airola

ASTHMA .....

HERBAL COMBINATIONS: (B R E) or (Breathe-Aid) and (ANTS Liquid Extract)
PHYSIOLOGIC ACTION: BRE or Breath-Aid effectively relieve symptoms associated with asthma, chest congestion and inflammation. Promotes free breathing, eliminates mucus and cleanses the body. ANTS Liquid Extract helps to relax bronchial spasms. It helps to cut mucus, and is helpful for chronic coughs.
SINGLE HERBS: Lobelia, Comfrey, Chlorophyll, Fenugreek, Mullein, and Nettle.
VITAMINS: A, B complex, B2, B3, B5, B6, B12, C, E, F, and Paba.
MINERALS: Manganese.
ALSO: Bee Pollen, honey, (honey will aid in clearing mucus out of the lungs.) Garlic, juice fast, vegetarian diet.
REFERENCES:
"How to Get Well"—P. Airola
"Nutrition Almanac"—J. Kirschmann
"Health Through God's Pharmacy"—M. Treben

ATHLETES FOOT .....

SINGLE HERBS: Caprinex (caprylic acid) and Pau d'Arco.
VITAMINS: Vitamin C powder (crystals) applied directly to affected area helps fungus infestation.
ALSO: Keep dry and out of shoes until infection clears.
REFERENCES:
"The Athletes Bible Glob Health

"The Fitness Formula" — S. Sokol

ATHLETIC INJURIES

HERBAL COMBINATION: (B F + C)
PHYSIOLOGIC ACTION: A special formula to aid in healing processes for torn cartilage's, sprained limbs, broken bones, multiple athletic injuries and associated swelling and inflammation.
SINGLE HERBS: White Oak Bark, Comfrey Root, Black Walnut Hulls, Lobelia and Skullcap.
VITAMINS AND MINERALS: A complete multi-one a day, (time released).
ALSO: Green-Lipped Mussel.
REFERENCES:
"The Athletes Bible - Glob Health
"The Fitness Formula" — S. Sokol

BACK PAIN .....

HERBAL COMBINATIONS: (Extress) (Kalmin Extract)
PHYSIOLOGIC ACTION: The herbs in these combinations help to relax muscles and reduce muscle tension. The Kalmin Extract has anti-spasmodic and anti-inflammatory qualities which are helpful in back pain caused by muscle strain.
SINGLE HERBS: Licorice, Valerian, and White Willow Bark.
VITAMINS AND MINERALS: Vitamin C and E, Calcium, Magnesium, Manganese.
AMINOS: DL-Phenylalanine and L-Tryptophan.
REFERENCES:
"How to Get Well"—P. Airola
"Global Herb Manual" — Zeke Fortisevn

BAD BREATH .....

SINGLE HERBS: Chlorophyll, Myrrh, Parsley, Peppermint, and Rosemary.

VITAMINS: A, B complex, B3, B6, C, and Paba.
MINERALS: Magnesium, and Zinc.
ALSO: Primadophilus.
REFERENCES:
"Vitamin Bible"—E. Mindell
"Halitosis"—M. Crag

BALDNESS . . . . .

SINGLE HERBS: Aloe Vera, Kelp, Primadophilus, Rosemary, Nettle, Yarrow, and Yucca
VITAMINS: A, B complex, B3, B5, B6, C, Biotin, Folic Acid, and Inositol.
MINERALS: Copper, Iodine, and Magnesium.
ALSO: L-Cysteine, L-Methionine, Protein, and Raw Thymus Glandular.
REFERENCES:
"Stop Hair Loss"—P. Airola
"Complete Natural Health Encyclopedia" - David Nyholt

BEE STINGS . . . . .

SINGLE HERBS: Echinacea, Pau d'Arco, and Yellow Dock Tea.
VITAMINS: B1 is a good insect repellent, and it creates a smell at the level of skin, that insects do not like. C — if already stung, use vitamin C to ease allergic reaction (acts as a natural antihistamine).
MINERALS: Calcium.
REFERENCES:
"Complete Natural Health Encyclopedia" - David Nyholt
"Natural Treatments & Remedies"—Global Health

BELCHING . . . . .
Refer to "Gas Intestinal" Page 25

BLADDER (IRRITABLE) . . . . .
Refer to Kidney and Bladder Page 32

BLEEDING GUMS . . . .
Refer to "Teeth and Gums" Page 46

BLOOD CLEANSER . . .

HERBAL COMBINATION: (Red Clover Combination)
PHYSIOLOGIC ACTION: Helps cleanse the blood of toxins, mucus, and infections thus helps improve and sustain overall good health; used for many years with very good results.
SINGLE HERBS: Red Clover, Chaparral, Dandelion, Garlic, and Burdock. *MINERALS:* Iron.
ALSO: Chlorophyll and Diulaxa tea.
REFERENCES:
"Herbally Yours"—P. Royal
"The Herb Book"—J. Lust
"Global Herb Manual"— Fortisevn
"Vitamin Bible"—E. Mindell

BLOOD CLOTS . . . . .
HERBAL COMBINATIONS: (Garlicin HC)
PHYSIOLOGIC ACTION: A comb- ination of herbs that help strengthen the heart while building and cleansing the arteries and veins.
SINGLE HERBS: Comfrey, Garlic, Golden Seal, Kelp, and Rose Hips.
VITAMINS: B complex (stress) C, E, Inositol, Choline, and Niacin.
MINERALS: Calcium, Magnesium, and Selenium.
ALSO: Evening Primrose Oil and Fish Oil.
REFERENCES:
"Herbally Yours"—P. Royal
"Blood Pressure"—Donsbach
"Complete Natural Health Encyclopedia" - David Nyholt
"Global Herb Manual" - Zeke Fortisevn
"Natural Treatments & Remedies"—Global Health

BLOOD PRESSURE (HIGH).....

HERBAL COMBINATION: (BP) (Cayenne-Garlic) (Garlicin HC)
PHYSIOLOGIC ACTION: BP improves overall blood circulation and tends to normalize high or low pressure to the body's normal level. Cayenne-Garlic and Garlicin HC lower blood pressure.
SINGLE HERBS: Cayenne, Garlic, Hawthorn, Kelp, Mistletoe, Valerian Root, and Yarrow.
VITAMINS: A, B Complex, B3, B5, B15, C, D, E, P, Inositol, Choline, and Lecithin.
MINERALS: Calcium, Magnesium, and Potassium.
REFERENCES:
"Herbally Yours"—P. Royal
"Complete Natural Health Encyclopedia" - David Nyholt
"Global Herb Manual"- Fortisevn

BLOOD PRESSURE (LOW).....

HERBAL COMBINATION: (B/P)
PHYSIOLOGIC ACTION: A time proven formula that improves overall blood circulation and tends to normalize high or low pressure to the body's normal level. Also reduces cholesterol build-up in the blood vessels. Helps relieve symptoms of cold and flu.
SINGLE HERBS: Garlic, Hawthorn, Siberian Ginseng, Kelp, Golden Seal Root, Ginger Root, and Spirulina,
VITAMINS: A, B Complex, B5, C, E, P, and Lecithin.
ALSO: EPA. and Salmon oil.
REFERENCES:
"Herbally Yours"—P. Royal
"Global Herb Manual"- Fortisevn
"Vitamin Bible"—E. Mindell
"Nutrition Almanac"—J. Kirschmann

BLOOD PURIFIER....
(General Detoxifier)

HERBAL COMBINATION: (Red Clover Combination)
PHYSIOLOGIC ACTION: This combination effectively aids the body's cleansing systems, especially the bloodstream. Should be included as a nutritional supplement in all chronic or degenerative conditions. Can be used with most detoxification programs.
SINGLE HERBS: Alfafa, Alfamax, Burdock, Chaparral, Echinacea, Devils Claw, Oregon Grape Root, Pau d' Arco, Red Clover, and Yellow Dock.
MINERALS: Iron, and Germanium.
REFERENCES:
"Herbally Yours"—P. Royal
"Global Herb Manual"- Fortisevn
"Health Through God's Pharmacy"—M. Treben

BOILS.....

HERBAL COMBINATION: (AKN)
PHYSIOLOGIC ACTION: Many skin diseases are often related to liver dysfunction. This herbal formula combines herbs which support the liver, and clean the blood.
FOR PAIN: Make a paste of wheat flour and honey, spread over area, and cover with cotton dressing.
SINGLE HERBS: Chaparral, Dandelion, Echinacea, Lobelia, Mullein, and Red Clover.
VITAMINS: A, C, E. Vitamin A may be applied locally.
MINERALS: Zinc (preventative).
REFERENCES:
"Natural Treatments & Remedies"—Global Health
"Health Through God's Pharmacy"—M. Treben

BONE, FLESH AND CARTILAGE.....

HERBAL COMBINATION: (BF + C)

PHYSIOLOGIC ACTION: A special formula to aid the body's healing processes involved with broken bones, athletic injuries, sprained limbs, and related inflammation and swelling. A tonic used after acute and chronic diseases to help rebuild the body.

SINGLE HERBS: Comfrey Root, Black Walnut, Lobelia, Skullcap, and White Oak Bark.

VITAMINS: A, C, and D.

MINERALS: Calcium, and Magnesium.

NOTE: Vitamin C and Calcium accelerate bone healing.

REFERENCES:
"The Athletes Bible" — Global Health
"The Fitness Formula" — S. Sokol
"Global Herb Manual"- Fortisevn

BOWEL CLEANSER.. (LOWER)

HERBAL COMBINATION: (Multilax #2) or (Naturalax #2)

PHYSIOLOGIC ACTION: Accelerates natural cleansing of the body and improves intestinal absorption by gentle evacuation of the bowels. It cleans out old, toxic fecal matter, mucus and encrustation's from the colon wall, and helps normalize the peristaltic action and rebuild the bowel structure. Use until the bowel is cleansed, healed, and functioning normally.

Warning: Do not take during pregnancy.

SINGLE HERBS: Cascara Sagrada, Golden Seal Root, Lobelia, Red Raspberry, and Senna.

VITAMINS: B complex.

ALSO: Flax seeds, Psyllium seeds, Whey Powder, Brewers Yeast, Yogurt, soaked Prunes and Figs, and Licorice tea.

REFERENCES:
"Colon Health"—Walker
"How to Get Well"—P. Airola
"Global Herb Manual"- Fortisevn
"Vitamin Bible"—E. Mindell

BREAST CANCER.....
Refer to "Cancer" Page 15

BREAST FEEDING...

SINGLE HERBS: Alfalfa, Blessed Thistle, Chlorophyll, Fennel, Red Raspberry, or Marshmallow (warm) will bring in good rich milk. Sage will help dry up the milk when the mother is ready to quit nursing.

VITAMINS: If baby has a cold, mother can take extra vitamin C.

CAUTION: A nursing mother should not take cleansing herbs as it may cause colic or diarrhea in the baby.

REFERENCES:
"Herbally Yours"—P. Royal
"Global Herb Manual"- Fortisevn

BREATHING DIFFICULTIES.....

HERBAL COMBINATIONS: (B R E) or (Breathe-Aid) (Fenu-Comf)

PHYSIOLOGIC ACTION: Effectively relieves irritation and promotes healing throughout the respiratory tract. Eliminates mucus, inflammation of the lungs, and helps relieve symptoms of coughs, colds, and bronchitis.

SINGLE HERBS: Comfrey Leaves, Lobelia, Marshmallow Root, and Mullein.

VITAMINS: C.

ALSO: Respa-Herb and Bee Pollen.

REFERENCES:
"Health Through God's Pharmacy"—M. Treben

BRIGHTS DISEASE ...

HERBAL COMBINATION: (KB)
PHYSIOLOGIC ACTION: Extremely valuable in healing and strengthening the kidneys, bladder, and genito-urinary area.
SINGLE HERBS: Alfalfa, Barberry Root, Catnip, Dandelion, Fennel, Ginger Root, Horstail, and Wild Yam..
VITAMINS: A, B complex, C, D, E, and Choline.
ALSO: Cranberry Juice, Propolis, Uratonic, and 3-Way Herb Teas.
REFERENCES:
"Complete Natural Health Encyclopedia" - David Nyholt
"Natural Treatments & Remedies"—Global Health

BRONCHITIS ....

HERBAL COMBINATION: (Fenu-Comf)
PHYSIOLOGIC ACTION: Helps relieve symptoms of coughs, colds, bronchitis, and helps eliminate mucus, congestion and inflammation from the lungs.
SINGLE HERBS: Comfrey, Eucalyptus, Lobelia, Chickweed Tea, Slippery Elm. Cayenne taken with Ginger cleans out the bronchial tubes.
VITAMINS: A, B12, C, and E.
MINERALS: A multi-mineral plus Zinc.
ALSO: Acidophilus-Liquid.
REFERENCES:
"Herbally Yours"—P. Royal

BRUXISM ....
Refer to "Teeth Grinding" Page 46

BURNING FEET ....
VITAMINS: B6.
MINERALS: Iron.
REFERENCES:
"How to Get Well"—P. Airola

BURNS ....

SINGLE HERBS: Aloe Vera, and Comfrey.
PHYSIOLOGIC ACTION: Aloe Vera is very good for burns, it may be used internally and externally. Some Aloe Vera preparations contain lanolin, which will intensify burns. Use a preparation without lanolin. Aloe Vera is especially good for acid burns.
VITAMINS: C, E, Paba. (Vit E applied directly to burn). Take vitamin C hourly-this may prevent infection from occurring.
MINERALS: Zinc.
ALSO: Ice, cold water, Paba cream, liquid honey, and Comfrey poultice.
REFERENCES:
"Herbally Yours"—P. Royal
"Aloe Vera Handbook"—M. Skousen
"Vitamin Bible"—E. Mindell
"Nutrition Almanac"—J. Kirshmann
"How to Get Well"—P. Airola

BURSITIS ....

HERBAL COMBINATIONS: (Rheum-Aid) (Cal-Silica) (Kalmin)
PHYSIOLOGIC ACTIONS: These herbal combinations contain herbs which exhibit anti-inflammatory and relaxing effects. Help to build nerve tissue, and relieve stiffness and pain.
SINGLE HERBS: Alfalfa, Chaparral, Comfrey. Mullein is often used as a poultice to give relief externally.
VITAMINS: A, B12, B Complex, C, E, and P.
MINERALS: Calcium and Magnesium.
ALSO: Peanut oil, and Alkaline diet.
REFERENCES:
"Herbally Yours"—P. Royal
"Vitamin Bible"—E. Mindel

CALCIUM DEFICIENCY...

HERBAL COMBINATION: Ca -T
PHYSIOLOGIC ACTION: This proven formula contains organic calcium, Silica and other tranquilizing minerals help prevent cramps. A natural way to calm nerves and aid sleep in addition to rebuilding the nerve sheath, vein, artery walls, teeth, and bones.
SINGLE HERBS: Comfrey Root, Horsetail, and Lobelia.
VITAMINS: D.
MINERALS: Calcium, Fem-Cal.
ALSO: Dark green leafy vegetables such as kale, mustard greens, collard greens, cabbage, broccoli, are rich sources of easily assimilated calcium. Foods such as lentils, almonds, and sesame seeds are other good sources.
REFERENCES:
"Calcium Bible"—P. Hausman
"Global Herb Manual"- Fortisevn
"Health Through God's Pharmacy"—M. Treben

CALCULUS.....
Refer to "Kidney and Bladder Stones" Page 32

CANCER.....
HERBAL COMBINATION: (Red Clover Combination)
PHYSIOLOGIC ACTION: This herbal combination contains herbs that are very similar to the Hoxey formula used to treat cancer. It is unique in that it cleanses and feeds the body.

Canaid herbal drink is similar, in nature and properties, to the famous Essiac treatment that has supposedly cured thousands of terminal patients.

The herb Pau d' Arco possesses antibiotic, tumor inhibiting, virus killing, anti-fungal and anti-malarial properties. Red clover, burdock and chaparral act as blood cleansers.
SINGLE HERBS: Bloodroot, Buckthorn Bark, Burdock, Chaparral, Cleavers, Garlic, Ginger, Ginseng, Golden Seal, Liquid Echinacea Extract, Pau d' Arco, Red Clover, Suma, Violet Leaves, and Yucca.
ALSO: There are various Chinese herbs which have been used successfully while treating cancer, Some of these herbs include: Reishi Mushroom, Astragalus, Ligustrum, Codonopsis, and Schizandra.
Research indicates that pancreatic and other enzymes are a vital part of a cancer program. It has also been noted that potassium is vital. Along with all the supplements, coffee enemas are important to cleanse the system and stimulate liver function.
VITAMINS: A, B3, B complex, C, E, Beta Carotene, and Digestive Enzymes.
MINERALS: Germanium, Magnesium, Potassium, and Selenium.
ALSO: Almonds, Apricot Pits, Red Beet Juice, Liver Extract, Brewers Yeast, Raw Food, Low Animal Protein, and Green Juices.
REFERENCES:
"Cancer, the Total Approach"—P. Airola
"Killing Cancer"—J. Winters
"Second Opinion"—B. Weed

CANDIDA ALBICANS
HERBAL COMBINATION: (Cantrol)
PHYSIOLOGIC ACTION: An excellent well balanced formula of herbs and supplements which balance the system while killing yeast. It includes caprylic acid and anti-oxidants for the control and eventual elimination of candida overgrowth.

SINGLE HERBS: Black Walnut, Caprinex, Garlicin, and Pau d'Arco.
VITAMINS: Biotin
ALSO: Linseed Oil, Candida Cleanse, Caprilic Acid, Primodophilus
REFERENCES:
"The Yeast Connection" — W. Crook, M.D.
"Candida Albicans" — L. Chaitow
"Candida Cookbook" — S. Rockwell

CANKER SORES ....

SINGLE HERBS: Burdock root tea, Goldenseal, and Pau d'Arco.
VITAMINS: A, B5, B12, B Complex, and large doses of C.
MINERALS: Iron.
ALSO: Avoid sugar and citrus fruits.

CARDIOVASCULAR DISEASE .....
Refer to Arteriosclerosis Page 9

CARPAL TUNNEL SYNDROME .....

SINGLE HERBS: Ginger Root Caps.
VITAMINS: B complex, B6, and C.
MINERALS: Calcium and Magnesium.
ALSO: Bromelain.
REFERENCES:
"Complete Natural Health Encyclopedia" - David Nyholt

CAR SICKNESS .....
Refer to "Motion Sickness" Page 36

CATARACTS .....

HERB COMPLEX: The following combinations are available by prescription only. - Cineraria Maritima, D3.

PHYSIOLOGIC ACTION: This product is a Homeopathic medicine and only available through your Homeopathic Doctor. Used regularly, this product will dissolve cataracts completely, after cataracts have disappeared use gencydo for minor inflammation.
HERBAL COMBINATION: (Herbal Eyebright Formula)
PHYSIOLOGIC ACTION: This herbal product contains valuable nutrients for the eyes. If taken regularly, in conjunction with a proper diet, cataracts are likely to dissolve.
SINGLE HERBS: Standardized Bilberry Extract.
VITAMINS: B2, and Riboflavin.
MINERALS: Copper, Manganese, Selenium, and Zinc.
ALSO: L-Lysine neutralizes viruses.
REFERENCES:
"Complete Natural Health Encyclopedia" - David Nyholt

CERVICAL DYSPLASIA .....

SINGLE HERBS: Bloodroot and Calendula.
VITAMINS: A, B complex, B6, B12, Folic Acid, and C.
MINERALS: Selenium and Zinc.
ALSO: Bitter Orange Oil, Bromelain, and Escarotic treatment.
REFERENCES:
"Natural Treatments & Remedies" — Global Health

CHARLEY HORSE ...
HERBAL COMBINATIONS: (BF & C)
PHYSIOLOGIC ACTION: This formula aids in the healing process for torn cartilage's, sprained limbs, broken bones, athletic injuries, and associated swelling and inflammation.

SINGLE HERBS: Comfrey, Horsetail, Oat Straw, Skullcap, and Yucca.
VITAMINS: B complex (stress), B1, B2, B5, C, D, and E.
MINERALS: Calcium, Magnesium, and Phosphorous.
ALSO: #12 tissue salts, Green-Lipid Mussel, Silica, Protein, and Unsaturated Fatty Acids.
REFERENCES:
"The Athletes Bible" — Global Health

CHICKEN POX . . . . .
HERBAL COMBINATION: (Fenu-Thyme) (ANT_PLG Syrup) (EchinaGuard)
PHYSIOLOGIC ACTION: Helps the body to resist infectious diseases and reduce fever.
SINGLE HERBS: Cayenne, Chickweed, Cleavers, Echinacea, Lobelia, and Red Clover.
ALSO: A bath con be made from bulk chickweed to alleviate itching. Chickweed ointment is also excellent for itching.
VITAMINS: Complete Multivitamin plus A, C, and E.
MINERALS: Multimineral plus Potassium and Zinc.
REFERENCES:
"Communicable Diseases"—L. Marks
"Herb Manual " — E. White

CIRCULATION . . . . .
HERBAL COMBINATIONS: (H Formula) (Ginkgold)
PHYSIOLOGIC ACTION: Contains herbs which strengthen the heart and builds the vascular system. When taken with Cayenne, it improves circulation, giving a warming sensation to the entire body.
ALSO: Cayenne strengthens the pulse rate and circulation while Black Cohosh slows it down.

SINGLE HERBS: Cayenne, Black Cohosh, Bayberry, Butchers Broom, Ginkgo, and Yarrow.
VITAMINS: A, B3, C, E, and Lecithin.
MINERALS: Calcium, Magnesium, and Potassium
REFERENCES:
"Herbally Yours"—P. Royal
"Global Herb Manual"- Fortisevn

CIRRHOSIS OF THE LIVER. . . . .
SINGLE HERBS: Barberry, Burdock, Celandine, Dandelion, Echinacea, Fennel, Garlic, Golden Seal, Hops, Milk Thistle, Red Clover, and Suma.
VITAMINS: A, B3, B9, B12, B complex, C, D, E, and K.
MINERALS: Magnesium, and Zinc.
ALSO: Carbohydrates, Coenzyme Q10, L-Carnitine, L-Glutathionine, L-Methionine, and Protein.
REFERENCES:
"Complete Natural Health Encyclopedia" - David Nyholt
"Natural Treatments & Remedies"—Global Health

COLD FEET . . . . .
HERBAL COMBINATION: (Cayenne extract)
PHYSIOLOGIC ACTION: Improves pulse rate and circulation giving a warming sensation to the entire body.
SINGLE HERBS: Cayenne, Bayberry, and Kelp.
VITAMINS: Vitamin E and Niacin.
MINERALS: A complete multi-mineral complex.
REFERENCES:
"Herbally Yours"—P. Royal
"Vitamin Bible"—E. Mindell

COLDS AND COUGHS . . . . .

HERBAL COMBINATIONS:
(Fenu-Thyme) (Garlic Syrup) (Loquat Syrup) (Garlicin CF)
PHYSIOLOGIC ACTION: These herbal syrups and combinations work to soothe the throat and lungs and act as expectorants and demulcents to cut and expel mucus from the lungs. Garlicin CF is a unique formula combining the natural benefits of Garlic with other herbs such as Echinacea, Vitamin C, bioflavanoids and Zinc.

COLDS AND FLU . . . .
(See Colds and Cough)

HERBAL COMBINATIONS:
(C+F) (Herbal Influence) (ANT-PLG Syrup)
PHYSIOLOGIC ACTION: Proven herbal formulas to help relieve symptoms of colds, flu, hoarseness, colic, cramps, sluggish circulation, beginning of fevers and germinal viral infections. Herbal Influence (formerly known as Herbal Composition) this formula was created by the early American herbalist, Samuel Thomson. It contains herbs which help with fever and nausea.
SINGLE HERBS: Cayenne, Red Clover, Raspberry Tea, Chaparral, Rose Hips, Garlic, Honey, and Golden Seal.
VITAMINS: A, B6, C, and P.
MINERALS: A Multi-mineral complex.
REFERENCES:
"Global Herb Manual"- Fortisevn
"How to Get Well"—P. Airola

COLD SORES . . . . .
(Herpes Simplex)

VITAMINS: Vitamin C with Vitamin P, and vitamin E oil applied directly.

MINERALS: Zinc.
ALSO: Lysine, and Primodophilus.
REFERENCES:
"Vitamin Bible"—E. Mindell

COLIC - (BABIES)

HERBAL COMBINATION:
(Catnip and Fennel Extract)
PHYSIOLOGIC ACTION: This formula works on minor spasms, acid stomach and gas. It also soothes indigestion and nerves. Excellent for children.
SINGLE HERBS: Catnip, Fennel, Camomile, Peppermint or any combination in a tea. Make teas very mild. No sugar. Check your own diet if nursing baby.
REFERENCES:
"Herbally Yours"—P. Royal

COLITIS . . . . .

SPECIFICS: Mucous Colitis is often associated with, and made worse by psychological stress. Emotional upset should be avoided. Various herbs with multiple properties must be used to address the complexity of this situation.
Single herbs to be used in combination: Bayberry, Camomile, Garlic, Reshi Mushroom, Valerian, and Wild Yam.
ALSO: Avoid citrus juices. Bananas are very soothing and healing in ulcerative colitis. Primadophilus is effective in stabilizing flora in lower bowel.
SINGLE HERBS: Alfalfa, Bayberry, Camomile, Caraway, Garlic, Peppermint, Reshi Mushroom, Plantain, Valerian, and Wild Yam.
VITAMINS: A, B6, B Complex, C, and E.
MINERALS: Calcium Lactate, Iron, Magnesiun, and Potassium.
REFERENCES:
"How to Get Well"—P. Airola

"Indian Herbology of North America"—A. Hutchens

CONSTIPATION.....

HERBAL COMBINATIONS: (Multilax #2) or (Naturalax #2) (Laxacil) (Naturalax 1) (Naturalax 3) (Aloelax Formula)

PHYSIOLOGIC ACTION: There are two forms of laxatives, stimulant and bulk forming. Stimulant laxatives encourage peristalsis of the bowel. This motion empties the intestinal tract of waste. Bulk forming laxatives absorb water and toxic wastes from the intestinal walls. The natural expansion triggers peristalsis, and pushes old fecal matter through the bowel. Both forms of laxatives have benefits.

Warning: Most laxatives should not be taken during pregnancy. Psyllium husks, however, are safe.

SINGLE HERBS: Aloe Vera, Cascara Sagrada, Psyllium, and Senna.

Babies: Licorice tea (made weakly). Nursing mothers can pass this one to the infant.

VITAMINS: A, B Complex, C, D. and E.

MINERALS: Calcium, Magnesiun, Potassium, and Zinc.

ALSO: Primadophilus

REFERENCES:
"Herbally Yours"—P. Royal
"Global Herb Manual" — Zeke Fortisevn
"Vitamin Bible"—E. Mindell
"How to Get Well"—P. Airola

COUGHS.....

HERBAL TONICS: Pie Pa Koa, Salus, Olbas, and Swiss herbal candy.

VITAMINS: A, B6, C, and P.

ALSO: Fenugreek Seed, Comfrey Leaves, Garlic, Honey, Rose Hips, fresh juice, short fasts, and Zinc Lozenges.

REFERENCES:
"The Miracle of Garlic"—P.Airola
"How to Get Well"—P. Airola
"Vitamin Bible"—E. Mindell
"Health Through God's Pharmacy"—M. Treben

CRADLE CAP.....

PHYSIOLOGICAL ACTION: Olive oil or vitamin E on the head and brush gently.

ALSO: A mild dandruff shampoo can be used.

REFERENCES:
"Herbally Yours"—P. Royal

CRAMPS.....
(Refer to "Leg Cramps" or "Menstrual Cramps" in Guide)

CROHN'S DISEASE..

SINGLE HERBS: Echinacea, Garlic, Golden Seal, Pau d'Arco, Rose Hips, and Yerba Mate.

VITAMINS: A, B12, B complex, and E.

MINERALS: A Complete Mineral Complex.

ALSO: Acidophlus, Aloe Vera, Essential fatty acids, and Protein.

REFERENCES:
"Complete Natural Health Encyclopedia" - David Nyholt
"Natural Treatments & Remedies"—Global Health

CROUP.....

HERBAL COMBINATIONS: (Breath aid) (BRE)

PHYSIOLOGIC ACTION: Helps to restore free breathing by opening up the bronchial passages. Effective for shortness of breath, tightness of chest, and wheezing associated with croup.

SINGLE HERBS: Comfrey, Echinacea tincture, Fenugreek, and Golden Seal.

VITAMINS: A, C, and E.

MINERALS: Zinc.

ALSO: Cod Liver Oil and Protein.
REFERENCES:
"Herbally Yours"—P. Royal
"Complete Natural Health Encyclopedia" - David Nyholt
"Global Herb Manual" Z Fortisevn

CYSTITIS .....
Refer to Kidney and Bladder Page 32

DEAFNESS .....
Refer to "Ear Infection" Page 22

DANDRUFF .....
SINGLE HERBS: Burdock, Chaparral, Red Clover, and Yarrow, (used as teas or rubbed on the head).
VITAMINS: A, B complex, B6, C, and E.
MINERALS: Selenium and Zinc.
ALSO: Unsaturated fatty acids.
REFERENCES:
"Back to Eden"—J. Kloss
"Stop Hair Loss"—P. Airola

DEPRESSION .....
HERBAL COMBINATIONS: (Ginseng, Gotu Kola Plus) (Adren-Aid)
PHYSIOLOGIC ACTION: These excellent formulas build zest, energy, stamina, mental alertness and reflex action. The herbs also help provide adrenal support which affect depression.
SINGLE HERBS: Bee Pollen, Cayenne, Damiana, Gotu Kola, St. John's Wort, Skullcap, Shitaki Mushroom, Siberian Ginseng, and Yucca.
VITAMINS: B3, B6, B12, B complex (stress), and lots of Vit C.
MINERALS: Multi-mineral Complex plus Calcium, Chromium, Magnesium, and Zinc.
ALSO: Tryptophan and L-Tyrosine
REFERENCES:
"Every Woman's Book"—P. Airola

"Amino Acids Book"—C. Wade
"Fighting Depression"—Ross
"the Athletes Bible" — Global Health

DERMATITIS .....
HERBAL COMBINATION: (AKN)
PHYSIOLOGIC ACTION: Many skin problems are related to liver dysfunction. This formula gives support to the liver, helps to cleanse the blood, and supplies nutrients for the skin.
SINGLE HERBS: Aloe Vera (on skin), Burdock, Cleavers, Dandelion, Evening Primrose, Garlic, Golden Seal, Pau d'Arco, and Yellowdock.
VITAMINS: A, B complex, B2, B3, B6, D, E, and Biotin B Complex.
MINERALS: Sulfur ointment, Zinc, and Potassium.
ALSO: Yu-ccan herbal drink.
REFERENCES:
"Nutrition Almanac"—J. Kirshmann

DIABETES .....
HERBAL COMBINATION: (PC)
PHYSIOLOGIC ACTION: An excellent formula to stimulate and restore natural functions, of the pancreas and spleen. Contains a natural form of insulin thus relieving most symptoms associated with diabetes.
SINGLE HERBS: Cayenne, Cedar Berries, Licorice Root, Mullein, Suma, Juniper and Uva Ursi.
VITAMINS: A, B complex, B1, B2, B6, B12, C, E, P, Choline, and Inositol.
MINERALS: Calcium, Chromium, Iron, Potassium, Magnesium, and Zinc.
ALSO: Protein and Proteolytic Enzymes.
REFERENCES:
"How to Get Well"—P. Airola

DIAPER RASH . . . . .

HERBAL OINTMENTS: (X-Itch ointment) (Derm-Aid Ointment)
SINGLE HERBS: Mullein Leaf, and Slippery Elm (used internally in juice or apply as paste).
ALSO: Vitamin E, Powdered Golden Seal, or Comfrey added to baby powder.
VITAMINS: Mom can take Vitamins A, B, and C.
REFERENCES:
"Herbally Yours"—P. Royal

DIARRHEA . . . . .

HERBAL COMBINATION: (Diarid) **PHYSIOLOGICAL ACTION:** This is a maximum-strength formula that relieves diarrhea and the pain and cramping that accompany it. The active ingredient is called Activated Attapulgite, a special kaolin substance with water absorbing abilities.
SINGLE HERBS: Blackberry Root, Red Raspberry, Slippery Elm, and Yucca.
ALSO: Nutmeg and Cloves for cramps.
VITAMINS: A, B complex, B1, B2, B3, B6, C, Folic Acid, and Choline.
MINERALS: Calcium, Chlorine, Iron, Magnesium, Potassium, and Sodium.
ALSO: Acidophilus, and Activated Charcoal.
Babies and Children: Slippery Elm enema, Red Raspberry tea, fresh apple juice, banana, carob.
REFERENCES:
"How to Get Well"—P. Airola
"Global Herb Manual"Z Fortisevn

DIGESTIVE DISORDERS . . . . .

HERBAL COMBINATIONS: (Multilax #2) or (Naturalax #2)

PHYSIOLOGIC ACTION: Helps intestinal gas, indigestion, heartburn, and stomach ache. Warm Peppermint tea, Cayenne, Papaya, or Aloe Vera can be taken with meals.
SINGLE HERBS: Aloe Vera, Chamomile, Cayenne, Comfrey leaves, Fennel, Ginger, Golden Seal, Licorice, Marshmallow Root, and Papaya.
VITAMINS: A, B3, B complex, and Biotin.
MINERALS: Copper, Dolomite, Iodine, Phosphorus, Potassium, and Zinc.
ALSO: Digestive Enzymes, Garlic, Bee Pollen, Calmus Root tea, Lactic Acid foods, Sweetish Bitters, Primodophlus and Yu-ccan herbal drink.
REFERENCES:
"Herbally Yours"—P. Royal
"Digestive Enzymes"—R.Passwater

DROPSY . . . . .

HERBAL COMBINATIONS: (KB)
PHYSIOLOGIC ACTION: KB acts as a mild diuretic to rid the body of excessive water.
SINGLE HERBS: Alfalfa, Buchu, Dandelion, tea, Juniper, Lobelia, Pau d' Arco tea, Safflower, Uva Ursi, and Yarrow.
VITAMINS: B1, B6, B complex, C, D, and E.
MINERALS: Calcium, Copper, and Potassium.
ALSO: L-Taurine, #9 and #11 Tissue Salts, Silicon, and Protein.
REFERENCES:
"Complete Natural Health Encyclopedia" - David Nyholt
"Global Herb Manual" — Zeke Fortisevn
"Natural Treatments & Remedies"—Global Health
"Nutrition Almanac"—J. Kirshmann

DRUG DEPENDENCY . . . . .

HERBAL COMBINATIONS:
(Adren Aid) (Red Clover Comb)
PHYSIOLOGIC ACTION: These herbal formulas provide support to the body while cleansing toxins. Red Clover Combination should be used with all detoxification programs.
SINGLE HERBS: Pau d'Arco, Camomile tea, Licorice Root, and Lobelia.
VITAMINS: B complex, and C.
MINERALS: Calcium, and Potassium.
ALSO: Tyrosine, Vitamins B, C, and E, alleviate depression, fatigue and irritability when dependent on cocaine, hashish, and marijuana.
Refer to: "Note in SMOKING" in this manual.
REFERENCES:
"Drugs & Beyond" - Global Health
"The Athletes Bible"—Global

DYSPEPSIA . . . . .
Refer Digestive Disorders Pg21

EAR INFECTION . . . .

HERBAL COMBINATIONS:
(Immun Aid) (B&B Extract) (EchinaGuard)
PHYSIOLOGIC ACTION:
ImmunAid boosts immunity, thereby helping with ear infections. EchinaGuard is a liquid. Echinacea extract is excellent for small children with ear infections. B&B Extract can be placed in the ear or taken internally. It is also used to aid poor equilibrium, and nervous conditions.
SINGLE HERBS: Blue Cohosh, Echinacea, Garlic Oil, Garlic, Mullein Oil, Mullein, Skullcap, and St. Johns Wort.

VITAMINS: A, B complex, and C.
MINERALS: Calcium and Zinc.
ALSO: Propolis, and Primadophilus. When combating ear infections, it is imperative to exclude allergen foods from the diet. This is particularly true of all dairy products.
REFERENCES:
"Back to Eden"—J. Kloss
"Global Herb Manual"Z Fortisevn

ECZEMA . . . . .

HERBAL COMBINATION:
(AKN)
PHYSIOLOGIC ACTION: When toxins are not properly eliminated from the body, they may surface through the skin creating eczema. This formula has been created to support liver and gall bladder function, to ensure toxins are filtered from the blood.
SINGLE HERBS: Aloe Vera, Chickweed, Evening Primrose Oil, Pau d'Arco, Red Clover, Thisilyn (Milk Thistle), and Yellow Dock.
VITAMINS: A, B complex, C, D, Paba, Biotin, Choline, and Inositol.
MINERALS: Magnesium, Sulfur Ointment, and Zinc Ointment.
ALSO: This condition is aggravated by food allergens such as dairy and wheat. These foods should be avoided. Powders and pastes should not be applied during acute or weeping stages. After acute stage passes, ointments and salves may be applied. Herbal ointments which contain Chickweed and Calendula are particularly helpful.
REFERENCES:
"How to Get Well"—P. Airola

EDEMA . . . . .

HERBAL COMBINATION: (KB)
PHYSIOLOGIC ACTION: K B acts as a mild diuretic to rid the body of excessive water.

SINGLE HERBS: Buchu, Dandelion tea, Juniper, Parsley, Safflower, Uva Ursi, and Yarrow.
VITAMINS: B1, B6, B complex, C, D, and E.
MINERALS: Calcium, Copper, and Potassium.
ALSO: #9, #11 tissue salts, Protein, and low sodium.

EMPHYSEMA .....

HERBAL COMBINATIONS: (Breath-Aid) (BronCare) (Garlicin CF)
PHYSIOLOGICAL ACTION: These natural formulas help to restore free breathing by dilating bronchial passages. They also offer nutritional support to the lungs.
SINGLE HERBS: Anise Seed Oil, Comfrey, Elecampane, Garlic, Lobelia, Mullein, and Swedish Bitters.
VITAMINS: A, B complex, C, D, E, Folic Acid.
ALSO: L-Cysteine, and L-Methionine,
REFERENCES:
"Stop Hair Loss"—P. Airola
"How to Get Well"—P. Airola

ENTEROBIASIS ...
Refer to "Parasites" Page 39

EPILEPSY .....

HERBAL COMBINATION: (B&B Tincture)
PHYSIOLOGICAL ACTION: The herbs in this formula have a beneficial effect on the autonomic nervous system. It helps to calm the nerves and relax the muscles.
ALSO: Avoid all refined sugars, completely eliminate all animal proteins, except milk as they rob body of magnesium and Vitamin B6 reserves. Eat lots of raw vegetables and fruit. Epileptics require plenty of fresh air, exercise and sound sleep.

SINGLE HERBS: Black-Cohosh, Horse Nettle, Hyssop, Irish Moss, Mistletoe, and Skullcap.
VITAMINS: A, B complex, Niacin, B6, B15, C, D, and E.
MINERALS: Calcium, Chromium, Iron, and Magnesium.
ALSO: Germanium, L-Taurine, L-Tyrosine, Proteolytic Enzymes, and Digestive Enzymes.
REFERENCES:
"Body Mind and Sugar"—E. Pezel
"Convulsive Disorders"—H. Keith
"How to Get Well"—P. Airola

EYE DISORDERS ....
HERBAL COMBINATION: (Herbal Eyebright Formula)
PHYSIOLOGIC ACTION: Extremely valuable in strengthening and healing the eyes. Aids the body in healing lesions and eye injuries.
Warning: If symptoms persist, discontinue use.
ALSO: The herb eyebright may be used as a wash for superficial inflammations of the eye.
SINGLE HERBS: Bilberry, and Eyebright.
VITAMINS: A, B1, B2, B3, B5, B6, C D, and E.
MINERALS: Calcium, Copper, Mangan- ese, Selenium, Magnesium and Zinc.
ALSO: Gyncydo and Protein.
REFERENCES:
"Herbally Yours"—P. Royal
"Vision Revised"—Donsbach

FATIGUE, STRESS, (Chronic) .....
HERBAL COMBINATIONS: (Adren Aid) (Echinacea Astragalus and Reshi Combination) (ImmuneAid) (Healthy Greens)
PHYSIOLOGIC ACTION: The herbs in these combinations work to support the adrenal glands and

act as a tonic boost to the immune system.

ALSO: Recent studies have shown that a combination of Evening Primrose Oil, and Fish Oil is very beneficial in combating chronic fatigue. The original study used a product called, "Efamol Marine." This product is not available in the United States nor Canada. It can be replicated by combining the individual Evening Primrose Oil capsules with Fish Oil, or Fish Liver Oil.

SINGLE HERBS: Astragalus, Cayenne, Echinacea, Siberian Ginseng, Ginseng, Gota Kola, Lobelia, Reshi Mushroom, and all deep green herbs such as Barley Grass, Chlorella, Spirulina, and Garlic.

VITAMINS: A, Ester C with Bioflavonoids, B complex (high potency), E, D, and Folic Acid.

MINERALS: Iron, Magnesium, Manganese, Potassium, Selenium, and Zinc.

ALSO: Canaid and Yu-ccan herbal drinks, Coenzyme Q 10, and Raw Thymus.

REFERENCES:
"Herbally Yours"—P. Royal
"Ginseng"—Donsbach

FATIGUE, (CHRONIC)

HERBAL COMBINATIONS: Recent studies have shown that a combination of Evening Primrose Oil, and Fish Oil is very beneficial in combating chronic fatigue. The original study called, "Efamol Marine." This product is not available in the United States nor Canada. It can be replicated by combining the individual Evening Primrose Oil capsules with Fish Oil, or Fish Liver Oil.

Other combinations include: AdrenAid, Echinacea Astragalus and Reshi Combination, ImmuneAid, & Healthy Greens.

PHYSIOLOGICAL ACTION: The herbs in these combinations work to support the adrenal glands and acts as a tonic boost to the immune system.

SINGLE HERBS: Astragalus, Echinacea, EchinaGuard Liquid Extract, Siberian Ginseng, Reshi Mushroom, all deep green herbs such as Barley Grass, Chlorella, Spirulina, and Garlic.

VITAMINS: Ester C with Bioflavonoids, B Complex, E, and D.

MINERALS: Calcium, Magnesium, Potassium, Selenium, and Zinc.

ALSO: CoQ 10, and Raw Thymus.

REFERENCES:
"The Athletes Bible" — Global
"The Fitness Formula" — S. Sokol

FATIGUE (GENERAL)

HERBAL COMBINATION: (Herbal UP) (Energizer) (AdrenAid)

PHYSIOLOGIC ACTION: These herbal formulas combine herbs which support the adrenals, tone the system, and offer stamina, and improve performance.

SINGLE HERBS: Siberian Ginseng, Gotu Kola, and Bee Pollen.

VITAMINS: Multivitamin, plus B Complex, B 12, and Vitamin C.

MINERALS: GTF Chromium, Potassium, Selenium, and Zinc.

REFERENCES:
"The Athletes Bible" — Global
"The Fitness Formula" — S. Sokol

FEVER-FLU COMPLAINTS . . . . .

HERBAL COMBINATIONS: (Fenu-Thyme) (Herbal Influence) (Immune Aid)

PHYSIOLOGIC ACTION: These effective formulas help to cleanse toxins, combat infections and inflammations especially in the lymphatic system. They give support to the immune system enabling the body to combat the illness.

VITAMINS: A, B complex, B3, C, E, and P.

MINERALS: Calcium, Phosphorus, Potassium, and Sodium.

ALSO: Canaid herbal drink, Propolis, Red Raspberry, Elder Flowers, Garlic, Rosehip, Golden Seal, Yarrow, Red Clover, #4 tissue salts.

Catnip and Peppermint together at onset of flu. Lemon or Grapefruit juice.

Babies and Children: Red Raspberry or Peppermint tea.

REFERENCES:
"The incurables"—Christopher
"Herbally Yours"—P. Royal

FLATULENCE . . . . .
Refer to Digestive Disorders Page 21

FOOD POISONING . .
SINGLE HERBS: Pau d' Arco.
VITAMINS: C and E.
MINERALS: Multi-mineral complex.
ALSO: Acidophlus, L-Cysteine, L-Methionine, and Fiber.
REFERENCES:
"Complete Natural Health Encyclopedia" - David Nyholt

FRIGIDITY . . . . .
HERBAL COMBINATIONS: (APH)
PHYSIOLOGIC ACTION: Stimulates male and female sexual impulses as well as strengthens and increases sexual power and helps fight fatigue.
SINGLE HERBS: Damiana, Ginkgo, Ginseng, and Goto Kola.
VITAMINS: E, Paba, Folic Acid, and Lecithin.

MINERALS: Calcium, Iodine, and Zinc.
ALSO: L-Arginine, L-Tyrosine, Proteolytic Enzymes, Melbrosia (for men), Bee Pollen, and Sesame Seeds.
REFERENCES:
"Complete Natural Health Encyclopedia" - David Nyholt
"Natural Treatments & Remedies"—Global Health

FUNGUS INFESTATIONS
(Athletes foot, thrush)
VITAMINS: A, B, C, and E.
ALSO: Primadophilus, Black Walnut, and Caprinex.
REFERENCES:
"Back to Eden"—J. Kloss

GAS INTESTINAL . . .
Intestinal gas is often the result of faulty digestion. (Digestive Disorders Page 21)
HERBAL COMBINATION: (LG)
PHYSIOLOGIC ACTION: Excellent formula for relieving intestinal gas, also cleanses liver and gall bladder.
SINGLE HERBS: Catnip, Ginger, Peppermint, and Horseradish are helpful for colon gas.
VITAMINS: B complex, B1, and B5.
ALSO: Eucarbon, Primadophilus, #8 tissue salts, and activated charcoal.
REFERENCES:
"Global Herb Manual"Z Fortisevn
"How to Get Well"—P. Airola

GASTRITIS . . . . .
SINGLE HERBS: Calamus, Chamomile, Dandelion, Marshmallow, Meadowsweet, and Swedish Bitters.
VITAMINS: A, B complex, B6, B12, C, D, E, and Lecithin.
MINERALS: Calcium and Iron.

ALSO: Diet and lifestyle influence this condition. It is important to avoid all food irritants such as spices and fiber. Avoid acidic foods such as tomatoes and citrus fruits. Stress reduction is important.
REFERENCES:
"Herbally Yours"—P. Royal
"Global Herb Manual"Z Fortisevn

GINGERVITIS . . . . .

SINGLE HERBS: Chamomile, Echinacea, Lobelia, Myrrh Gum, and White Oak Bark.
VITAMINS: A, B complex, C, D, P, Niacin, and Folic Acid.
MINERALS: Calcium, Copper, Magnesium, Manganese, Phosphorus, Potassium, Silicon, Sodium, and Zinc.
ALSO: Coenzyme Q10, Protein, and Unsaturated Fats.
REFERENCES:
"Complete Natural Health Encyclopedia" - David Nyholt
"Natural Treatments & Remedies"—Global Health

GLAND INFECTIONS

HERBAL COMBINATION: (IGL)
PHYSIOLOGIC ACTION: Combats infection and reduces inflammation from the body, especially the lymphatic system, ears, throat, lungs, breasts and organs of the body.
VITAMINS: C
ALSO: Propolis, Golden Seal, Saw Palmetto, and Echinacea.
REFERENCES:
"Glandular Extracts"—Donsbach
"Herbally Yours"—P. Royal
"Health Through God's Pharmacy"—M. Treben

GLAND PROBLEMS . .

HERBAL COMBINATIONS: (GL) (IF)
PHYSIOLOGIC ACTION: Effective for swollen lymph nodes

and in helping the body fight glandular weakness and infections.
SINGLE HERBS: Alfalfa, Calendula, Echinacea, Golden Seal, Lobelia, Mullein, Saw Palmetto, and Skullcap.
VITAMINS: A, B5, B Complex, C, and E.
MINERALS: Calcium, Magnesium, and Potassium.
ALSO: Multi Glandulars, Primrose Oil.
REFERENCES:
"Glandular Extracts"—Donsbach
"Herbally Yours"—P. Royal

GLAUCOMA . . . . .
(Hypertension of the eye)

SPECIFICS: It is believed that restoration of vision lost due to nerve degeneration cannot occur. However the vitamins and herbs listed can be effective in controlling and preserving the remaining sight.
HERBAL SUPPLEMENTATION: Herbal Eyebright Formula, KB, Bilberry, and Extress.
PHYSIOLOGIC ACTION: These herbs work to restore balance to the system. They supply nutrition to the eye, while helping to remove excessive fluids and toxins. They also help to reduce problems associated with stress.
NOTE: It is important to keep in contact with your doctor while working with this serious eye problem.
HERB COMBINATION: (Eyebright Comb)
VITAMINS: A, B2, B5, B Complex, C, D, and E.
MINERALS: A good comprehensive muti- mineral formula.
ALSO: Germanium.
REFERENCES:
"How to Get Well"—P. Airola
"Health Bulletin"—Feb 15, 1964

GOITER .....

SINGLE HERBS: Kelp is an excellent source of iodine.
VITAMINS: A, B6, B complex Choline, C, and E..
MINERALS: Calcium and Iodine.
ALSO: Protein.
REFERENCES:
"Natural Treatments & Remedies"

GONORRHEA .....

SINGLE HERBS: Echinacea, Golden Seal, Pau d' Arco, and Suma.
VITAMINS: B complex and K.
MINERALS: Zinc.
ALSO: Acidophilus, Coenzyme Q10, Germanium, and Protein.
REFERENCES:
"Complete Natural Health Encyclopedia" - David Nyholt

GOUT .....

HERBAL COMBINATION: (Yucca AR), (Rheum Aid) (Yu-ccan herbal drink)
PHYSIOLOGIC ACTION: These formulas are effective in helping to reduce swelling and inflammation in body joints and connective tissues. Also helps relieve stiffness and pain.
SINGLE HERBS: Burdock, Dandelion Root, Lobelia, Stinging Nettle, Safflower, Pau d'Arco tea, and Yucca.
VITAMINS: A, B complex, B5, C, and E.
MINERALS: Calcium, Magnesium, and Potassium.
ALSO: Primadophilus. Diet plays a vital function in the treatment of this malady. Foods containing Uric Acids, such as meat, and rich pastries need to be avoided. All purine-rich foods need to be avoided, such as anchovies, herring, sardines, mushrooms, mussels, and liver.

REFERENCES:
"Athletes Bible" — Global Health
"The Fitness Formula" — S. Sokol

GRIPPE .....
Refer to "Colds and Flu" Pg. 18

GYNECOLOGICAL PROBLEMS .....

HERBAL COMBINATION: (Fem-Mend)
PHYSIOLOGIC ACTION: Menstrual regulator, tonic for genito-urinary system. Helpful for severe menstrual discomforts. Acts as an aid in rebuilding a malfunctioning reproductive system (Uterus, ovaries, fallopian tubes, etc.)
SINGLE HERBS: Aloe Vera, Blessed Thistle, Comfrey Root, Garlic, Ginger, Golden Seal Root, Red Raspberry, Slippery Elm Bark, Uva Ursi, and Yellow Dock Root,
VITAMINS: A, B Complex, C, E.
MINERALS: Multi-mineral.
REFERENCES:
"Global Herb Manual" Z Fortisevn
"Fitness Formula" — Steve Sokol

HARDENING OF THE ARTERIES .....
Refer to "Arteriosclerosis" Pg. 9

HAY FEVER .....

HERBAL COMBINATIONS: (HAS Original and Fast Acting Formulas) (Allergy Care)
PHYSIOLOGIC ACTION: These herbal formulas contain a natural extract of Pseudoepheda, in a base of herbs, which help to restore free breathing without causing drowsiness. HAS original is for those sensitive to Ephedra.
SINGLE HERBS: EchinaGuard Nettle tea, Elder Flowers, Eye Bright, Golden Seal, Golden Rod, Swedish Bitters, and Yarrow

VITAMINS: A, B complex, B6, Ester C with Bioflavaniods, and E.
ALSO: Coenzyme Q10, Bee pollen granules or tablets. Pollen-rich unprocessed raw honey.
REFERENCES:
"Vitamin Bible"—E. Mindell
References listed for "Allergies".

HEADACHE . . . . .

HOMEOPATHIC COMBINATION: (Tension Headache Formula)
SINGLE HERBS: Chamomile and Feverfew.
VITAMINS: A, B1, B2, B3, B6, B12, B complex, C, D, E, and F.
MINERALS: Calcium, Magnesium, Potassium, and Zinc.
ALSO: Acidophilus, and Q10.
REFERENCES:"
Complete Natural Health Encyclopedia" - David Nyholt
"Natural Treatments & Remedies"—Global Health

HEART . . . . .

HERBAL COMBINATIONS: (H) (Garlicin HC)
PHYSIOLOGIC ACTION: Promotes elasticity of arteries. Helps eliminate cholesterol, also aids in rebuilding the heart, strengthening and regulating the beat of the heart, and improving circulation in general.
SINGLE HERBS: Barberry, Cayenne, Garlic, Hawthorn Berries, Lobelia, and Shepherds Purse.
VITAMINS: A, B1, B5, B15, C, D, E, Lecithin, Biotin, Inositol, Choline, and Folic Acid.
MINERALS: Calcium, Copper, Iodine, Iron, Magnesium, and Potassium.
REFERENCES:
"Heart and Vitamin E"—Shute
"How to Get Well"—P. Airola

HEART BURN . . . . .

HERBAL COMBINATION: (Motion Mate)
SINGLE HERBS: Chamomile, Chewable Papaya, Meadowsweet, and Marshmallow Root.
ALSO: Digestive enzymes (especially Pancreatic enzymes), bone meal, and primadophilus

HEMORRHOIDS . . . .

HERBAL COMBINATION: (Yellow Dock Formula)
PHYSIOLOGIC ACTION: Effective formula for hemorrhoids, colitis and blood purifier. Also revitalizes prolapsed uterus, kidneys and bowl.
SINGLE HERBS: Butchers Broom, Collinsonia Root, Horsechestnut, Lobelia, Stone Root, and Yellow Dock.
VITAMINS: A, B6, B Complex, C, E, P, and Vit E oil.
MINERALS: Multi-mineral plus Calcium.
ALSO: Bulk forming laxatives such as Laxacil, or Psyllium seed husks are recommended to take pressure from the colon. Combination "Hem Relief" ointment, Pile ointment and suppositories or Circu Caps Witch Hazel Compresses.
REFERENCES:
"How to Get Well"—P. Airola
"Vitamin Bible"—E. Mindell

HIATAL HERNIA . . . .

SINGLE HERBS: Aloe Vera Juice, Comfrey, Goldenseal, and Red Clover.
VITAMINS: A, B12, B Complex, and C.
MINERALS: Multi-Mineral plus Zinc
ALSO: Pancreatin, Papaya, and Proteolytic Enzymes.

REFERENCES:
"Complete Natural Health Encyclopedia" - David Nyholt
"Natural Treatments & Remedies"—Global Health

HORMONE REGULATION.....

FEMALE HERBAL COMBINATIONS: (MP) or (Change-O-Life)
PHYSIOLOGIC ACTION: This herbal formula is effective in regulating hormonal imbalance. Its greatest benefit is for the relief of the symptoms of menopause. Also good for youth during puberty.
SINGLE HERBS: Blessed Thistle, Damiana, Dong Quai, Mistletoe, and Vitex Agnus Castus
MALE HERB COMBINATION: (APH)
PHYSIOLOGIC ACTION: Stimulates sexual impulses, strengthens and increases sexual power. Help eliminate fatigue and increases longevity.
SINGLE HERBS: Damiana, Fo-Ti, Gota Kola, Sarsaparilla Root, Saw Palmetto, and Siberian Ginseng.
MINERALS: Potassium.
REFERENCES:
"Herbally Yours"—P. Royal
"Every Woman's Book"—P. Airola
"Health Through God's Pharmacy"

HORMONE IMBALANCE.....
Refer to "Menopause" Page 35

HOUSEMAID'S KNEE.....

HERBAL COMBINATIONS: (Rheum- Aid) (Cal-Silica) (Kalmin)
PHYSIOLOGIC ACTION: These herbal combinations contain herbs which exhibit anti-inflammatory and relaxing effects. Help to build nerve tissue and relieve stiffness and pain.
SINGLE HERBS: Alfalfa, Chaparral, and Comfrey.
VITAMINS: A, B12, B complex, C, E, and P.
MINERALS: Calcium Magnesium.
ALSO: Alkaline diet, Coenzyme Q10, Germanium, and Protein supplements.
REFERENCES:
"Complete Natural Health Encyclopedia" - David Nyholt
"Natural Treatments & Remedies"

HYPERACTIVITY....

HERBAL COMBINATION: (Wild Lettuce and Valerian Extract)
PHYSIOLOGIC ACTION: This excellent formula is a natural sedative. Promotes overall calming of the nerves and restores a sense of control and balance without causing drowsiness.
ALSO: Ginkgo or Ginkgold. Although this herb is often used to promote circulation, it also has a positive effect on the nervous system, Used in conjunction with the following single herbs, and with a balanced, chemical free diet, good results can be expected.
SINGLE HERBS: Evening Primrose Oil Lobelia, Oat Extract, Skullcap, St. Johns Wort, Valerian, and Wild Lettuce.
VITAMINS: High potency B vitamins, B3, B5, B6, and C.
NOTE: Yeast free B vitamins may be required if yeast intolerance is present.
MINERALS: High doses of all minerals.
Note: avoid all foods with artificial flavoring and coloring. Processed foods should be eliminated from the diet. Foods which contain natural salicylates such as apples, and oranges need to be avoided.

REFERENCES:
"The Hyperactive Child"—Barnes and Colquhoun.

HYPERTHYROIDISM .

HERBAL COMBINATIONS: (GL) (IF)
PHYSIOLOGIC ACTIONS: Effective for swollen lymph nodes and in helping the body fight glandular weakness and infections.
SINGLE HERBS: Alfalfa, Calendula, Echinacea, Golden Seal, Lobelia, Mullein, Saw Palmetto, and Skullcap.
VITAMINS: A, B5, B Complex (stress), C, and E.
MINERALS: Calcium, Magnesium, and Potassium.
ALSO: Multi Glandulars and Primrose Oil.
REFERENCES:
"Herbally Yours"—P. Royal
"Natural Treatments and Remedies"—Global Health

HYPOGLYCEMIA . . . .

HERBAL COMBINATIONS: (HIGL) (AdrenAid)
PHYSIOLOGIC ACTION: Stimulates the adrenals and the pancreas to help restore sugar levels, helps correct glandular imbalances, eliminates toxins, assists the body in handling stress conditions and promotes a feeling of well being.
Note: Some people who have hypoglycemia cannot handle Golden Seal, as it tends to lower the blood sugar. Safflower is good to take before exercise.
VITAMINS: A, B3, B complex, C, E, and Folic Acid.
MINERALS: Magnesium, and Potassium.
ALSO: Bee Pollen, Juniper, Glyco-lite, Acidophilus. Low animal protein, small meals high in natural complex carbohydrates.

REFERENCES:
"Hypoglycemia"—P. Airola
"How to Get Well"—P Airola
"Vitamin Bible"—E. Mindell

HYPOTHYROIDISM . .

HERBAL COMBINATION: (T)
PHYSIOLOGIC ACTION: An excellent formula to help revitalize and promote healing of the thyroid glands, thus restoring metabolism balance.
VITAMINS: A, B1, B5, C, D, E, and F.
MINERALS: Calcium, Magnesium, and Potassium.
ALSO: Brewers Yeast, Essential Fatty Acids, Protein, and Thyroid Glandular.
REFERENCES:
"Glandular Extracts"—Donsbach
"Herbally Yours"—P. Royal
"Health Through God's Pharmacy"—M. Treben
"Global Herb Manual"Z Fortisevn
"Natural Treatments & Remedies"—Global Herb Manual
"The Complete Natural Health Encyclopedia"—D. Nyholt

IMPETIGO . . . . .

HERBAL COMBINATIONS: (Red Clover Combination) (Yellow Dock Formula) (AKN)
PHYSIOLOGIC ACTION: These herbal formulas effectively aid the body's cleansing systems thus helps eliminate ulcers of the skin, impetigo etc.
SINGLE HERBS: Echinacea, Licorice Root and Red Clover.
VITAMINS: A, C, D, E. Vitamin A and E applied topically. Vitamin A is necessary for the health of the skin tissue, and vitamins C, D, and E, may be helpful in aiding the skin in its recovery from impetigo.
REFERENCES:
"Back to Eden"—J. Kloss
"Nutrition Almanac"

IMMUNE DEFICIENCY . . . . .

HERBAL COMBINATION: (Echina Guard)
PHYSIOLOGIC ACTION: Stimulates the immune response systems. Especially helpful in rebuilding the body during convalescence and as a preventative.
SINGLE HERBS: Echinacea Root, Chaparral, Korean White Ginseng, Pau d' Arco, Rosemary, and Golden Seal Root.
VITAMINS: A Multi-vitamin plus B6, B12, C, and E.
MINERALS: A strong complete multi - time release
ALSO: Canaid herbal Drink, L-Cysteine, L-Methionine, L-Lysine, L-Ornithine, Propolis and Primadophilus.

IMPOTENCE . . . . .

HERBAL COMBINATION: APH.
PHYSIOLOGIC ACTION: Stimulates male and female sexual impulses as well as strengthens and increases sexual power and helps fight fatigue.
VITAMINS: E, Paba, Folic Acid, and Lecithin.
MINERALS: Zinc, Iodine, and Calcium.
ALSO: Melbrosia (for men), Tropical Impulse tea, and Loving Mood.
ALSO: Sesame Seeds, Ginseng, Damiana, high quality vegetable oil, fertile eggs, and raw milk.
REFERENCES:
"Herbally Yours"—P. Royal
"How to Get Well"—P. Airola

INDIGESTION . . . . .
Refer to Digestive Disorders Page 21

INFERTILITY . . . . .

SINGLE HERBS: Dong Qui and Gotu Kola.

VITAMINS: A, B6, B Complex, and E.
MINERALS: A Complete Mineral Complex.
ALSO: Astrelin, Gerovital H3, L-Tyrosine, Proteolytic Enzymes, and Raw Ovarian Concentrate.
REFERENCES:
"Natural Treatments & Remedies"
"The Complete Natural Health Encyclopedia"—D. Nyholt

INFLUENZA . . . . .
Refer to Colds and Flu Page 18

INSOMNIA . . . . .

HERBAL COMBINATIONS: (E-Z Sleep) (Silent Night)
PHYSIOLOGIC ACTION: Soothing mild relaxant. Promotes natural restful and refreshing sleep.
SINGLE HERBS: Catnip, Hops, Skullcap, Pau d'Arco, and Valerian Root.
VITAMINS: B1, B3, B, B6, D, and E.
MINERALS: Calcium, Iron, Magnesium, and Potassium
ALSO: Taheebo, Protein, and Tryptophan.
REFERENCES:
"Amino Acids Book"—C. Wade

INTESTINAL PARASITES . . . . .
Refer to "Parasites" Page 39

JAUNDICE (NON INFECTIOUS) .

HERBAL COMBINATION: (LG)
PHYSIOLOGIC ACTION: This herbal combination helps to correct malfunctioning of the liver and gall bladder. It is a liver detoxifier, and a bile stimulant.
SINGLE HERBS: Birch Leaves, Dandelion, Fennel, Horse Tail, Irish Moss, and Rose Hips.

VITAMINS: A, B6, C, D, and E.
MINERALS: Calcium, Magnesium and Phosphorus.
ALSO: Lecithin, Protein, and Unsaturated fatty acids.
REFERENCES:
"How to Get Well"—P. Airola
"The Nature Doctor"—A. Vogel

JET LAG . . . . .

SPECIFIC: Siberian ginseng, taken on a regular bases for about a week before the trip, seems to have a balancing effect on the system, lessening the effects of Jet Lag. A good vitamin supplement is also helpful. **SINGLE HERBS:** Gota kola, Korean Ginseng.
VITAMINS: Stress B Complex, Multi-Vitamin, C, and E.
MINERALS: Multi-mineral complex.
REFERENCES:
"Vitamin Bible"—E. Mindell

KIDNEY AND BLADDER . . . . .

HERBAL COMBINATION: (KB)
PHYSIOLOGIC ACTION: Extremely valuable in healing and strengthening the kidneys, bladder and genito-urinary area. Useful to stop bed wetting, but is a diuretic when congestion of the kidneys is indicated. Helps remove bladder, uterine and urethral toxins.
Warning: Intended for occasional use only. May cause green-yellow discoloration of urine.
VITAMINS: A, B complex, C, D, E, and Choline.
MINERALS: Calcium, Magnesium, and Potassium.
ALSO: Cranberry juice, Propolis, Uratonic, Watermelon, 3-way herb teas, and other Diuretic tablets
REFERENCES:
"Own Your Own Body"—S. Malstom

"Lets Get Well"—A. Davis
"Every Woman's Book"—P. Airola
"How to Get Well"—P. Airola

KIDNEY FUNCTIONS . . . . .

SINGLE HERBS: Garlic and Parsley.
PHYSIOLOGIC ACTION: Promotes urine flow and strengthens kidneys. Also revitalizes and strengthens liver and spleen.
ALSO: Propolis, Cranberry juice, 3-way herb teas, and Uratonic.
Refer to Kidney and Bladder in this manual.
REFERENCES:
"Diets to Help Cystitis"—McCutcheon
"Back to Eden"—J. Kloss
"Vitamin Bible"—E. Mindell

KIDNEY - BLADDER STONES . . . . .

HERBAL COMBINATION: (PR)
PHYSIOLOGIC ACTION: PR comb helps dissolve kidney stones. PR helps keep kidneys flushed out (toxins and buildup of waste and sediments). Juniper keeps kidneys flushed out. Parsley acts as a diuretic. Magnesium helps prevent stones from forming. Thyme helps prevent buildup and dissolves stones if already present.
SINGLE HERBS: Corn silk, Dandelion, Juniper, Parsley, Thyme, and Uva Ursi.
VITAMINS: A, B2, B5, B6, C, E, F, and Choline.
MINERALS: Magnesium, and Potassium.
ALSO: Apple Juice, Lemon Juice, and Marshmallow.
REFERENCES:
"Vitamin Bible"—E. Mindell
"How to Get Well"—P. Airola
"Health Through God's Pharmacy"—M. Treben

LABOR AND DELIVERY . . . . .

Red Raspberry is essential during labor. It coordinates the uterine contractions often making labor shorter.
REFERENCES:
"Herbally Yours"—P. Royal

LAXATIVES . . . . .

HERBAL COMBINATION:
(Multilax #1) or (Naturalax #1)
PHYSIOLOGIC ACTION: Helps relieve minor constipation.
Warning: Do not use when abdominal pain nausea or vomiting are present. Frequent or prolonged use of preparation may result in dependence on laxatives.
ALSO: Vita Cleansing Tea, Swiss Kriss, Metab Herb, Psyllium Husks, Flaxmeal, Super D Tea. Drink lots of pure water to flush system.
REFERENCES:
"How to Get Well"—P. Airola
"Health Through God's Pharmacy"—M. Treben

LEG CRAMPS . . . . .
(Charley Horse)

HERBAL COMBINATION: (Ca-T)
PHYSIOLOGIC ACTION: Effectively clams nerves and aids sleep in addition to rebuilding the nerve sheath, vein and artery walls.
SINGLE HERBS: Comfrey Herb, Horsetail Grass, Oat Straw, and Skullcap.
VITAMINS: B complex, B5, C, D, and E.
MINERALS: Calcium, Magnesium and Phosphorus.
ALSO: #12 tissue salts
REFERENCES:
"Calcium Bible"—P. Hausman
"Vitamin Bible"—E. Mindell

LEG ULCERS . . . . .

HERBAL COMBINATION: (H Formula) (Ginkgold)
PHYSIOLOGIC ACTION: Strengthens the heart and builds the vascular system.
SINGLE HERBS: Cayenne, Bayberry, Butchers Broom, Ginkgo, and Yarrow.
VITAMINS: A, B3, B12, C, and E.
MINERALS: Calcium, Iron, Magnesium, and Potassium.
ALSO: Coenzyme Q10, Germanium
REFERENCES:
"Herbally Yours"—P. Royal

LEUKEMIA . . . . .

SINGLE HERBS: Pau d'Arco, Swedish Bitters, and Nettle.
VITAMINS: B complex, B12, C, and E.
MINERALS: Copper, Iron, and Zinc.
Refer to "Cancer" in the manual
REFERENCES:
"Nutrition Almanac"—J. Kirschmann

LEUKORRHEA . . . .

HERBAL COMBINATION:
(Cantrol)
PHYSIOLOGIC ACTION: An excellent well-balanced formula of herbs and supplements which balance the system while killing yeast.
SINGLE HERBS: Black Walnut, Caprinex, Garlic, Pau d' Arco, and Yucca.
VITAMINS: A, B Complex, Biotin, D, and E.
MINERALS: Calcium and Magnesium.
ALSO: Yu-ccan Herbal Drink, Linseed Oil, Candida Cleanse, Caprilic Acid, and Primadophilus.
REFERENCES:
"Herbally Yours"—P. Royal

"Natural Treatments & Remedies"
"The Complete Natural Health Encyclopedia"—D. Nyholt

LIVER and GALLBLADDER

HERBAL COMBINATION: (LG)
PHYSIOLOGIC ACTION: Helps the cleansing of the liver and gall bladder, restores new energy to these organs. Also can be taken to relieve intestinal gas.
SINGLE HERBS: Bayberry Root, Catnip, Fennel Seed, Ginger Root, and Peppermint.
VITAMINS: A, B1, B2, B6, Choline, Niacin, Pantothenic Acid, C, and E.
MINERALS: Copper and Sulfur for the Liver. Magnesium and Sulfur for the Gallbladder.
ALSO: Acidophlis, Carrot juice, Calamus Root tea, Chlorophyll, and all green drinks.
REFERENCES:
"The Master Cleanser" — S. Burroughs
"Global Herb Manual"Z Fortisevn
"Health Through God's Pharmacy"—M. Treben

LIVER DISORDERS ..

HERBAL COMBINATIONS: (Thisilyn) — (Milk Thistle Extract)
PHYSIOLOGIC ACTION: Protects liver. Anti-oxidant quality prevents free radical damage in the liver.
SINGLE HERBS: Dandelion & Horsetail.
VITAMINS: A, B Complex, B1, B2, B3, B6, C, E, Choline, and Lecithin.
ALSO: Digestive Enzymes, and Primadophilus.
REFERENCES:
"How to Get Well"—P. Airola
"Nutrition Almanac"—J. Kirschmann

LOWER BOWEL PROBLEMS .....

HERBAL COMBINATIONS: (Multilax #2) or (Naturalax #2)
PHYSIOLOGIC ACTION: Accelerates natural cleansing of the body and improves intestinal absorption by gentle evacuation of bowls. Cleans out old toxic fecal matter, mucus and encrustation's from the colon wall and helps normalize the peristaltic action and rebuild the bowel structure. Use until the bowel is cleansed, healed and functioning normally.
SINGLE HERBS: Calamus Root, Golden Seal Root, Lobelia, Red Raspberry, Eucarbon, and Yucca..
VITAMINS: A Muiti-vitamin plus a B Complex.
MINERALS: A strong Multi-mineral Complex.
ALSO: Yu-ccan herbal drink, Flax Seeds, Psyllium Seeds, and Figs.
REFERENCES:
"Colon Health"—Dr. N. Walker
"Health Through God's Pharmacy"—M. Treben

LUMBAGO .....
Refer to "Back Pain" Page 10

MELANOMA .....

SINGLE HERBS: Kelp and Pau d' Arco.
VITAMINS: A, B Complex, B12, Niacin, Folic Acid, C, and E.
MINERALS: A strong Multi-mineral plus Calcium, Magnesium, and Potassium.
ALSO: Coenzyme Q10, Germanium, L-Cysteine, L-Methionine, L-Taurine, Essential Fatty Acids, Primadophilus, Proteolytic Enzymes and Raw Glandular Complex with extra Raw Thymus
REFERENCES:
"Glandular Extracts"—Donsbach

"Natural Treatments & Remedies"
"The Complete Natural Health
Encyclopedia"—D. Nyholt

MEMORY AID . . . . .

HERBAL COMBINATIONS:
(SEN) or (Remem)
PHYSIOLOGIC ACTION: This
formula contains remarkable
rejuvenating properties that
nourish the brain cells and tissues
and improves their ability to
perform mental functions.
SINGLE HERBS: Cayenne,
Ginkgo, Gotu Kola, Korean
Ginseng, and Lobelia.
VITAMINS: Choline, and
Lecithin. **MINERALS:** Multi-
mineral complex.
REFERENCES:
"Mental Alertness"—Donsbach
"Vitamin Bible"—E. Mindell

MENINGITIS . . . . .

SINGLE HERBS: Catnip and
Garlic.
VITAMINS: Multi-vitamin plus A,
C, and D.
MINERALS: A high potency
mineral complex, plus Calcium,
and Zinc.
ALSO: Germanium, Protein, and
Raw Thymus.
REFERENCES:
"Natural Treatments & Remedies"
"The Complete Natural Health
Encyclopedia"—D. Nyholt

MENOPAUSE . . . . .

HERBAL COMBINATIONS:
(Change-O-Life) or (MP)
PHYSIOLOGIC ACTION: For
both male and female health to
the pancreas, pituitary and other
glandular areas and maintains a
healthy hormone balance in the
body, especially during puberty
and menopause.
Warning: not intended for use
during pregnancy

SINGLE HERBS: Black Cohosh,
Blessed Thistle, Licorice Root,
Sarsaparilla, and Siberian Gin-
seng,
VITAMINS: A, B complex, B3, C,
D, and E.
MINERALS: Calcium, magnesium,
Potassium, and Selenium.
ALSO: Melbrosia, Damiana,
Germanium, Quan Yin, and Gin-
seng.
REFERENCES:
"Every Woman's Book"—P. Airola
"Vitamin Bible"—E. Mindell

MENSTRUATION . . . .

HERBAL COMBINATIONS: (FC)
or (FEM-MEND)
PHYSIOLOGIC ACTION: Helps
regulate the menstrual cycle, relieve cramps, bloating and vaginitis, ease inflammation of the
vagina and uterus, and
strengthen and regulate the kidneys, bladder and uterus areas.
Beneficial for all female and
uterine complaints.
Warning: Do not use this
combination while taking estrogen
or oral contraceptives.
SINGLE HERBS: Red Raspberry,
and Uva Ursi.
VITAMINS: B complex, B6, C, E,
and Iodine.
REFERENCES:
"Every Woman's Book"—P. Airola
"PMS Book"—Wade

MIGRAINE HEADACHES . . . . .

PHYSIOLOGIC ACTION: Camomile will prevent migraine headaches. Feverfew reduces fever.
Feverfew has been historically
used for chills and pain that
accompany fever. Because of its
anecdotal claims for migraine suf-
fers, it is presently being researched at the London Migraine
Clinic.

SINGLE HERBS: Camomile, & Feverfew.
VITAMINS: B3, B5, B12, B Complex, C, F, Paba, and Niacin.
MINERALS: Calcium, Magnesium, and Potassium.
ALSO: Unsaturated fatty acids.
REFERENCES:
"Feverfew Your Headache may be Over"—Hancock
"Global Herb Manual"Z Fortisevn
"Herbally Yours"—P. Royal
"How to Get Well"—P. Airola

MONONUCLEOSIS ..

VITAMINS: A, B complex, B1, B2, B5, B6, C, Biotin, and Choline.
MINERALS: Potassium.
ALSO: Canaid herbal drink, Germanium, Raw thymus, Raw Glandular Complex, and Protein.
REFERENCES:
"Natural Treatments & Remedies"
"Vitamin Bible"—E. Mindell

MORNING SICKNESS ....

SINGLE HERBS: Red Raspberry or Peppermint Tea often overcomes nausea. Alfalfa, Catnip, & Ginger tea may also be helpful. Sometimes small frequent meals instead of a larger one is beneficial.
VITAMINS: A Multi-vitamin plus B6, C, and K.
ALSO: Avoid cigarette smoke, alcohol, white sugar, refined carbohydrates, coffee, and other stimulants.
Note: Morning sickness may be due to either an intolerance or a deficiency.

MOTION SICKNESS .

HERBAL COMBINATION: (Motion Mate)
PHYSIOLOGIC ACTION: In a recent university study ginger root caps proved more effective than either a drug or placebo at controlling motion induced nausea, also queasy travelers have found taking B complex at night and just before the trip is most effective.
SINGLE HERBS: Ginger Root Caps.
VITAMINS: B complex plus B6.
ALSO: Charcoal tablets.
REFERENCES:
"Vitamin Bible"—E. Mindell
"Original Herb Formulas"L. Griffin

MOUTH SORES .....
(Canker, Thrush, Pyorrhea)

SINGLE HERBS: Aloe Vera, Golden Seal, Myrrh, Red Raspberry, and White Oak Bark.
VITAMINS: A, B2, B3, B12, B Complex, C, and E..
MINERALS: Iron, Magnesium, Phosphorus, and Zinc.
ALSO: Chlorophyll, Lysine, and Primadophilus.
REFERENCES:
"Bee Medicine"—Uccusic
"Healing Power of Chlorophyll"—Jensen

MULTIPLE SCLEROSIS .....

SINGLE HERBS: Evening Primrose Oil, Kelp, Oat Extract, Skullcap, and St.John's Wort.
VITAMINS: B complex, B1, B2, B3, B5, B6, B12, C, E, F, Inositol, and Lecithin.
MINERALS: Calcium, Copper, Iron, Magnesium, Manganese, Selenium, and Zinc.
ALSO: Bonemeal, Coenzyme Q10, Germanium, L-Leucine, L-Isoleucine, L-Valine, Protein, and Digestive Enzymes.
REFERENCES:
"How to Get Well"—P. Airola
"Nutrition Almanac"—J. Kirschmann

MUMPS .....
HERBAL COMBINATION: (ANT-PLG)
PHYSIOLOGIC ACTION: An effective formula that helps cleanse toxins and reduce infection. This combination is a natural aid in fighting contagious diseases.
SINGLE HERBS: Bayberry Root Bark, Echinacea, Ginger Root, Lobelia, and Mullein.
VITAMINS: A, B Complex, C, E.
MINERALS: A complete multi complex.
ALSO: Germanium and Acidophilus.

MUSCLE INJURIES ..
Refer to Athletic Injuries P. 10

MUSCULAR DYSTROPHY .....
SINGLE HERBS: Saw Palmetto.
VITAMINS: A, B complex, B3, B5, B6, B12, C, E, and Choline.
MINERALS: Potassium.
ALSO: Protein and Unsaturated fatty acids.
REFERENCES:
"How to Get Well"—P. Airola
"Nutrition Almanac"—J. Kirschmann

MYOCARDIAL INFARCTION .....
HERBAL COMBINATION: (Garlicin HC)
PHYSIOLOGIC ACTION: Strengthens the heart, cleanses arteries and veins, and builds the vascular system.
SINGLE HERBS: Cayenne, Comfrey, Evening Primrose Oil, Fish Oil, Garlic, Golden Seal, and Rose Hips.
VITAMINS: B Complex, C, E, Niacin, Inositol, and Choline.

MINERALS: Calcium and Magnesium.
ALSO: Coenzyme Q10, L-Carnitine, L-Cysteine, L-Methionine, Multidigestive Enzymes, DMG, Fish Oils, and Vegetable Oils.
REFERENCES:
"Natural Treatments & Remedies"
"Complete Natural Health Encyclo pedia"—D. Nyholt

NAUSEA - VOMITING
HERBAL COMBINATION: (Herbal Influence)
PHYSIOLOGIC ACTION: Contains herbs which help with fever and nausea.
SINGLE HERBS: Cayenne, Chaparral, Garlic, Raspberry, Red Clover, Rose Hips, Golden Seal.
VITAMINS: A, B6, C, and P.
MINERALS: Magnesium.
REFERENCES:
"Global Herb Manual"Z Fortisevn
"The Complete Natural Health Encyclopedia"—D. Nyholt

NERVOUS DISORDERS .....
(Tension, Anxiety)
HERBAL COMBINATIONS: (Calm-aid) or (Ex stress comb)
PHYSIOLOGIC ACTION: A proven formula that is soothing, strengthening and healing to the whole nervous system to relieve nervous tension and rebuild the nerve sheaths. Excellent aid for insomnia, chronic nervousness and stress-related conditions.
SINGLE HERBS: Evening Primrose Oil, Hops, Mistletoe, Skullcap, and Valerian.
VITAMINS: B complex, B1, B2, B3, B5, B6, and C.
MINERALS: Calcium, Iodine, Iron, Magnesium, Phosphorus, Potassium, Silicon, and Sodium.

REFERENCES:
"Stress Without Distress"—Selye
"Stress"—Donsbach

NEURITIS . . . . .

SPECIFICS: The best treatment for neuritis is to make sure the patient gets optimum nutrition.
SINGLE HERBS: Black Cohosh, Lobelia, Lady Slipper, Skullcap, and Valerian Root.
VITAMINS: B1, B2, B6, B12, Niacin and Pantothenic acid.
MINERALS: A strong Multi-mineral plus Calcium and Magnesium.
ALSO: Lecithin, Protein, and Proteolytic Enzymes.
REFERENCES:
"Lets Get Well"—A. Davis
"Nutrition Abstracts"—R. Ropert

NIGHT BLINDNESS .

HERBAL COMBINATION:
(Herbal Eyebright Formula)
PHYSIOLOGIC ACTION:
Extremely valuable in strengthening and healing the eyes. Aids the body in healing lesions and eye injuries.
Warning: If symptoms persist discontinue use.
SINGLE HERBS: Bilberry and Eyebright.
VITAMINS: A Multi-vitamin complex plus A, B1, B2, B3, B5, B6, C, D, and E.
MINERALS: Calcium, Copper, Manganese, Magnesium, Potassium, Selenium, and Zinc.
ALSO: Gyncydo and Protein.
REFERENCES:
"Herbally Yours"—P. Royal
"Global Herb Manual"Z Fortisevn
"Natural Treatments & Remedies"
"The Complete Natural Health Encyclopedia"—D. Nyholt

NOCTURIA . . . . .

HERBAL COMBINATION: (KB)

PHYSIOLOGIC ACTION:
Valuable in healing and strengthening the kidneys, bladder, and genito-urinary area.
SINGLE HERBS: Alfalfa, Barberry Root, Catnip, Dandelion, Fennel, Ginger Root, Goldenrod, Horsetail, Uva Vrsi, and Wild Yam.
VITAMINS: A, B Complex, C, D, E, and Choline.
MINERALS: Calcium, Magnesium, and Potassium.
ALSO: Digestive Enzymes, Lecithin, and 3 Way Herb Teas.
REFERENCES:
"Natural Treatments & Remedies"

OBESITY . . . . .

HERBAL COMBINATIONS:
(SKC) or (Herbal Slim)
PHYSIOLOGIC ACTION: This effective formula cleanses the bowels and eliminates excess water. Helps control appetite, dissolves excess fat, reduces tension, stress and anxiety associated with dieting.
SINGLE HERBS: Chickweed, Hawthorn Berries, Kelp, Licorice Root, Papaya Leaves, and Saffron.
VITAMINS: B2, B5, B6, B12, B complex, C, E, Choline, Folic Acid, Inositol, and Lecithin.
MINERALS: Calcium, Magnesium, and Phosphorus.
ALSO: Yu-ccan herbal drink, Protein, and Unsaturated fatty acids.
REFERENCES:
"Nutrition Almanac"—J. Kirschmann
"The Athletes Bible" — Global Health
"The Fitness Formula" — Steve Sokol

OSTEOARTHRITIS . .

HERBAL COMBINATION:
(Rheum- Aid) (Yucca - AR)

PHYSIOLOGIC ACTION: Helps the body reduce or eliminate swelling and inflammation in the joints and connective tissue.
SINGLE HERBS: Alfalfa, Black Cohash, Burdock, Cayenne, Celery Seed, Chaparral, Devil's Claw, Valerian Root, and Yucca.
VITAMINS: Niacin, B5, B6, B12, B Complex, C, D, E, F, and P.
MINERALS: A strong Multi-Mineral Plus Calcium, and Magnesium.
ALSO: Cod Liver Oil, Green Magma, Aqua Life, Seatone, and Bromelain.
REFERENCES:
"Herbally Yours"—P. Royal
"Natural Treatments & Remedies"—Global Health
"The Complete Natural Health Encyclopedia"—D. Nyholt

OSTEOPOROSIS . . . .

SINGLE HERBS: Feverfew, Horsetail, and Oatstraw.
VITAMINS: B12, C, D, and E.
MINERALS: Calcium, Copper, Fluoride, Magnesium, and Phosphorus..
ALSO: L-Arginine, L-Lysine, Protein, Multidigestive Enzymes with Betaine Hydrochloride, and Proteolytic Enzymes.
REFERENCES:
"Natural Treatments & Remedies"—Global Health
"The Complete Natural Health Encyclopedia"—D. Nyholt

PAIN . . . . .
(HEADACHES, Tension)

HERBAL COMBINATION: (A-P)
PHYSIOLOGIC ACTION: Helps relieve pain in any part of the body. A natural way to ease chronic pain, headaches, childbirth after-pains, aching teeth, nervous tension, spasms and intestinal gas.

SINGLE HERBS: Pau d'Arco.
MINERALS: Calcium.
ALSO: DLPA (amino acid), Lobelia, and Pau d'Arco.
REFERENCES:
"Diets to Help Headaches"—Nightingale
"The Athletes Bible" — Global

PANCREAS . . . . .

HERBAL COMBINATION: (PC)
PHYSIOLOGIC ACTION: Helps eliminate mucus and sedimentation, arrest infection, and stimulate and restore the natural functions of the pancreas. Also used for blood-sugar problems and healing the spleen.
SINGLE HERBS: Dandelion, Golden Seal, Juniper Berries, and Uva Ursi.
VITAMINS: A, B complex, C, E, Choline, and Inositol.
MINERALS: Chromium, Potassium and Zinc.
ALSO: Coenzyme Q10, Germanium, lecithin, Proteolytic Enzymes, and Raw Pancreas Concentrate.
REFERENCES:
"Glandular Extracts"—Donsbach
"How to Get Well"—P. Airola

PARASITES . . . . .

HERBAL COMBINATIONS: (Para-X) (Para-VF)
PHYSIOLOGIC ACTION: Useful in destroying and eliminating parasites, such as worms. Also helps relieve many kinds of skin problems. The Para-VF is liquid and is useful for children and the elderly who cannot swallow capsules.
Warning: Do not use during pregnancy.
SINGLE HERBS: Black Walnut, Garlic, Pumpkin Seeds, Sage, Swedish Bitters and Wormwood.
VITAMINS: Folic Acid.

CHILDREN: Camomile tea, or raisins soaked in Senna tea for older children may be helpful.
REFERENCES:
"The Miracle of Garlic"—P.Airola
"Herbally Yours"—P. Royal

PARKINSON'S DISEASE .....

SPECIFICS: A low protein diet of raw organic foods is best for patients with Parkinson's Disease.
SINGLE HERBS: Ginseng, Damiana, and Cayenne
VITAMINS: B complex, plus B2, B6, C, and E.
MINERALS: Calcium Lactate, and Magnesium.
ALSO: Brewer's yeast, Lecithin, Multi-digestive Enzymes, L-Glutamic Acid, and L-Tyrosine.
REFERENCES:
"New Breed of Doctor"—A. Nittler
"Ann. Rev. Med." 22: 305 — G. Cotzais

PEPTIC ULCERS ...

HERBAL COMBINATION: (Myrrh- Gold Seal Plus)
SINGLE HERBS: Golden Seal, Myrrh, Pau d' Arco, Red Raspberry, Slippery Elm Bark, Valerian, and White Oak Bark.
VITAMINS: A, B2, B5, B6, B12, B Complex, C, D, E, P, Choline, and Folic Acid.
MINERALS: Calcium, Magnesium, and Zinc.
ALSO: Acidophilus, Adrenal Glandular Extract, Bioflavonoids, Bromelain, and Glutamine.
REFERENCES:
"Natural Treatments & Remedies"—Global Health
"The Complete Natural Health Encyclopedia"—D. Nyholt

PHLEBITIS .....

HERBAL COMBINATIONS: (H Formula) (Garlicin HC)

PHYSIOLOGIC ACTION: The herbs in these combinations are known to strengthen and support the cardiovascular system. Supplementing the body with niacin (B3), may be useful to help prevent clot formation. Vitamin C can help strengthen the blood vessel walls. Some research indicates that vitamin E may dilate the blood vessels, thus discouraging the formation of varicose veins and phlebitis.
SINGLE HERBS: Ginkgo, Horse Chestnut and Yarrow.
VITAMINS: B complex, B3, C, and E.
MINERALS: Multi-mineral Complex.
REFERENCES:
"Nutrition Almanac"—J. Kirschmann

PINK EYE .....

SINGLE HERBS: Hot compresses made from Chamomile or Fennel tea may be helpful for irritation.
VITAMINS: A, B2, B6, B Complex, Niacin, C, and D.
MINERALS: Calcium, Magnesium, Phosphorus, and Zinc.
REFERENCES:
"Back to Eden"—J. Kloss
"Nutrition Almanac"—J. Kirschmann
"Herbally Yours"—P. Royal
"Natural Treatments & Remedies"—Global Health
"The Complete Natural Health Encyclopedia"—D. Nyholt

PINWORMS .....
Refer to "parasites" Page 39

PNEUMONIA .....

HERBAL COMBINATIONS: (Garlicin CF) (Herbal Influenza)
SINGLE HERBS: Boneset, Comfrey, EchinaGuard, Euca-

lyptus, Fenugreek, Licorice, and Mullein.
VITAMINS: A, B complex, Ester C with Bioflavonoids, E, K, and P.
MINERALS: Zinc.
REFERENCES:
"Back to Eden"—J. Kloss
"Herbally Yours"—P. Royal
"Nutrition Almanac"—J. Kirschmann

POOR CIRCULATION.....
Refer to "Circulation" Page 41

PREMENSTRUAL SYNDROME (P.M.S.).
Refer to "Menstruation" Page 35

PRE-NATAL PREPARATION.....
HERBAL COMBINATION: (Healthy Greens)
PHYSIOLOGIC ACTION: A complete combination of vitamins and minerals containing digestive aids to ensure proper assimilation.
SINGLE HERBS: Blessed Thistle, Chamomile, Chlorella, Lobelia, and Red Raspberry,
VITAMINS: A, B Complex, B12, C, D, and E.
MINERALS: Multi-mineral Complex plus Calcium, Magnesium, and Phosphorus.
ALSO: Bone Meal, Brewer's Yeast, and Kelp.
REFERENCES:
"Herbally Yours"—P. Royal
"Pregnancy"—Donsbach
"Every Woman's Book"—P. Airola

PROLAPSUS.....
HERBAL COMBINATION: (Yellow dock Combination)
PHYSIOLOGIC ACTION: Helps revitalize a prolapsed uterus, kidneys, and bowel, it also has been

proven effective for hemorrhoids, colitis, and as a good purifier.
SINGLE HERBS: Black Walnut, Calendula, Marshmallow Root, Mullein, White Oak Bark, and Yellow Dock.
REFERENCES:
"Health Through God's Pharmacy"—M. Treben
"Every Woman's Book"—P. Airola

PROSTATE and KIDNEY.....
HERBAL COMBINATION: (PR)
PHYSIOLOGIC ACTION: This formula helps cleanse sedimentation and arrest infection in the prostate and dissolve kidney stones to restore these glands to the natural functions.
SINGLE HERBS: Cayenne, Bee Pollen, Golden Seal, Juniper Berries, Siberian Ginseng, and Uva Ursi.
ALSO: ProActive is an herbal extract of Saw Palmetto.
VITAMINS: A, B complex, B6, C, E, and F.
MINERALS: Calcium, Magnesium, and Zinc.
PROSTATE SPECIFICS: Also regularity in sexual habit, lots of walking and other exercise.
REFERENCES:
"Health Through God's Pharmacy"—M. Treben
"Kidney Disorders"—H. Clements

PSORIASIS.....
HERBAL COMBINATIONS: (AKN) (Evening Primrose) (Thisilyn)
PHYSIOLOGIC ACTION: The above herbs taken in combination has a dramatic effect on this disorder.
SINGLE HERBS: Chickweed, Dandelion, Goldenseal, Lobelia, Skullcap, St. Johns Wort, and Yellow Dock.

VITAMINS: A, B complex, C, D, E, Folic Acid, and Lecithin.
MINERALS: Calcium, Magnesium, Sulfur Ointment, and Zinc.
ALSO: Diet and stress are key factors in this skin disorder. Certain allergen foods need to be completely avoided. Dairy and wheat are especially harmful in many instances. Fat should be kept to a minimum.
REFERENCES:
"How to Get Well"—P. Airola
"Nutrition Almanac"—Kirschmann
"Indian Herbology"—A. Hutchens

PYORRHEA . . . . .

SINGLE HERBS: Golden Seal, & Myrrh.
PHYSIOLOGIC ACTION: Use these powders on tooth brush, or make a tea, which is one teaspoon of each the Golden Seal and Myrrh, in one pint of boiling water. Steep. Rinse mouth and gargle with it freely, also, brush gums with the tea.
VITAMINS: A, B1, B2, B6, B12, C, D, and E. Rub the gums morning and evening with vitamin E.
MINERALS: Calcium, Magnesium, and Zinc.
REFERENCES:
"Back to Eden"—J. Kloss
"Nutrition Almanac"-Kirschmann

QUINSY . . . . .

HERBAL COMBINATION: (IF) (IGL)
PHYSIOLOGIC ACTION: Effective formulas that help cleanse toxins, combat infections, and heal the lymphatic system.
SINGLE HERBS: Bayberry Root, EchinaGuard, Enchinacea, Ginger Root, and Pau d' Arco.
VITAMINS: A complete multi-complex.
ALSO: Canaid herbal drink.

REFERENCES:
"Nutrition Almanac"—Kirschmann
"Natural Treatments & Remedies"
"The Complete Natural Health Encyclopedia"—D. Nyholt

RHEUMATIC FEVER . . . . .

SINGLE HERBS: Birch Leaves, Catnip, Dandelion, Fenugreek, Garlic, Lobelia, Thyme, and Pau d' Arco.
VITAMINS: A complete multi-complex plus A, B2, B6, C, D, and E.
MINERALS: Zinc
ALSO: Canaid herbal drink, Bioflav- onoids, Coenzyme Q10, and Germanium.
REFERENCES:
"Back to Eden"—J. Kloss
"Indian Herbalogy of North America"—A. R. Hutchens
"Natural Treatments & Remedies"
"The Complete Natural Health Encyclopedia"—D. Nyholt

RHEUMATISM . . . . .

HERBAL COMBINATIONS: (Yucca-AR) or (Rheum-Aid)
PHYSIOLOGIC ACTION: Excellent formulas for relieving symptoms associated with bursitis, calcification, gout, rheumatoid arthritis, rheumatism and osteoarthritis. It helps to reduce or eliminate swellings inflammation in joints, connective tissues and relieves stiffness and pain.
SINGLE HERBS: Alfalfa, Chaparral, Cayenne, Fennel, Garlic, Pau d'Arco, Red Clover, Red Raspberry and Yucca.
VITAMINS: B complex, B5, B15, C, and E.
MINERALS: Calcium, Magnesium phosphorus, Potassium, and Zinc.
ALSO: Yu-ccan herbal drink Digestive Enzymes, and Hydrochloric Acid.

REFERENCES:
"Folk Medicine"—Crest
"Back to Eden"—J. Kloss
"How to Get Well"—P. Airola

RINGING IN EARS ..
Refer to "Tinnitus" Page 46

RINGWORM .....
HERBAL COMBINATION:
(Black Walnut Extract)
SINGLE HERBS: Black Walnut, Golden Seal, Pau d'Arco. Rub skin with black walnut extract, Apple Cider Vinegar or Castor Oil, several times a day.
VITAMINS: A, B Complex, and C.
MINERALS: Zinc.
ALSO: Germanium and Unsaturated Fatty Acids.
REFERENCES:
"How to Get Well"—P. Airola
"Herbally Yours"—P. Royal

ROUNDWORMS .....
HERBAL COMBINATION:
(Para-X) (Para-VF)
PHYSIOLOGIC ACTION: Para-X is useful in destroying and eliminating parasites. Para-VF is a liquid and is used for children and the elderly who cannot swallow capsules.
SINGLE HERBS: Black Walnut, Garlic, Pumpkin Seeds, and Wormwood.
VITAMINS: Folic Acid.
ALSO: Swedish Bitters.
REFERENCES:
"Nutrition Almanac"—J. Kirschmann
"Natural Treatments & Remedies"—Global Health
"The Complete Natural Health Encyclopedia"—D. Nyholt

SCIATICA .....
HOMEOPATHIC REMEDY:
(Injury and Backache Formula)

PHYSIOLOGIC ACTION: For natural symptomatic relief of pain and discomfort.
SINGLE HERBS: Pau d' Arco.
VITAMINS: B1, B12, B Complex, D, and E.
MINERALS: Multi-mineral.
REFERENCES:
"Natural Treatments & Remedies"
"The Complete Natural Health Encyclopedia"—D. Nyholt

SCURVY .....
SINGLE HERBS: Kelp and Yucca.
VITAMINS: A, B Complex, C, and D.
MINERALS: Calcium, Iron, and Magnesium.
ALSO: Yu-ccan herbal drink and Protein.
REFERENCES:
"Nutrition Almanac"—J. Kirschmann
"Global Herb Manual"Z. Fortesvn
"Natural Treatments & Remedies"—Global Health
"The Complete Natural Health Encyclopedia"—D. Nyholt

SEIZURES .....
Refer to "Epilepsy" Page 23

SENILITY .....
HERBAL COMBINATIONS:
(SEN) or (Remem)
PHYSIOLOGIC ACTION: An excellent combination to nourish the brain cells, tissues and improves their ability to perform mental functions.
SINGLE HERBS: Dandelion, Ginkgo, Ginseng, Gotu Kola, Licorice, and Yellow Dock.
VITAMINS: A, B3, B complex, C, and E.
MINERALS: Choline and Zinc.
ALSO: Coenzyme Q10, Germanium, Lecithin, and Protein.

REFERENCES:
"Antioxidants"—Passwater
"Herbally Yours"—P. Royal

SHINGLES . . . .
(Herpes Zoster)
PHYSIOLOGIC ACTION: B vitamins are necessary for the proper functioning of the nerves. Vitamins A and C promote healing of skin lesions, and heavy doses of vitamin C can limit infection of lesions.
VITAMINS: A, B complex, C, and D.
MINERALS: Calcium, and Magnesium
ALSO: L-Lysine and Protein.
REFERENCES:
"Nutrition Almanac"J.Kirschmann

SINUS PROBLEMS . .
HERBAL COMBINATIONS: (HAS) (Zand Decongest Herbal Formula) (Garlicin CF)
SINGLE HERBS: Comfrey, Elderberry, Eyebright, Fenugreek, and Golden Seal.
VITAMINS: A, B complex, B5, C, and E.
MINERALS: Potassium and Zinc.
ALSO: Bee Pollen, Coenzyme Q10, Garlic, Germanium, Protein, and Proteolytic Enzymes.
REFERENCES:
"Diets to Help Catarrh"A. Moyle

SKIN . . . . .
(Bites, Stings, and Poisons)
PHYSIOLOGIC ACTION: Echinacea was used by the plains Indians to lessen the effects of poisonous bites. EchinaGuard would be very beneficial. Take large doses of vitamin C and Calcium. Use vitamin E topically to reduce pain.
REFERENCES:
"How to Get Well"—P. Airola

SKIN . . . . .
SINGLE HERBS: Hautex.
PHYSIOLOGIC ACTION: To work from within to encourage skin secretion, effective for acne, blackheads, pimples, itch and rash.
VITAMINS: A, B complex, E, C, and Rosehips.
ALSO: Efamol, Whey Powder, and Acidophilus

SKIN BLEMISHES . . .
HERBAL COMBINATION: AKN.
PHYSIOLOGIC ACTION: Diulaxa tea helps cleanse the bloodstream. Pimples, blackheads, and other superficial skin eruptions, and more serious conditions such as boils, carbuncles, dermatitis, eczema, and pleuritis will be eliminated when the blood has been cleansed.
VITAMINS: A, B2, B3, B5, B6, C, F, P, Biotin, and Paba.
MINERALS: Iron, Silicon, and Sulfur.
ALSO: Whey Powder, and Brewers Yeast.
REFERENCES:
"Diets to Help Acne"—A. Moyle

SKIN CANCER . . . . .
Refer to "Melanoma" Page 34

SKIN PROBLEMS . . . .
1. *Dry Skin* — Chamomile, Dandelion, Licorice, Oat Extract, Evening Primrose Oil, Vitamin A, B complex, C, Aloe Vera, Add Herbal oils to bath (Lavender oil is very nice)
2. *Itchy Skin* — Chickweed, Calendula, Elder, Yarrow, vegetable oil daily, apple cider vinegar to bath. X-Itch ointment is also very effective.
3. *Oily Skin* — Vitamin B complex, Liver, and Rosemary.

4. **Scars** — Vitamin E orally and topically.
5. **Stretch marks** — Vitamin E, B complex, B5, C, Aloe Vera, Zinc, and Carnation oil.
6. **Sunburn** — B vitamins, Paba, C, E, Calcium, Zinc, and Aloe Vera.
7. **Wrinkles** — Vitamins A, B complex, E, Zinc, Selenium, and Almond oil.

REFERENCES:
"Secrets of Natural Beauty" Castleton
"Swedish Beauty Secrets"P. Airola
"How to Get Well"—P. Airola

SMOKING . . . . .

HERBAL COMBINATIONS:
(Milk thistle extract) or (Thisilyn)
PHYSIOLOGIC ACTION: The herbal combination decreases the desire for tobacco and protects the liver from the negative effects of smoking. Vitamins and minerals should be taken to rebuild the nutritional system after a juice fast. The juice fast cleanses the accumulated poisons from the body, thus eliminating the physiological dependence.
Note: Tobacco, alcohol, caffeine and other drug "cravings" are brought about by a physiological body dependence on the poison which develops during prolonged use. The addicts blood poison level must remain at a certain level at all times. As the poison level drops, there is a "desire" to take in more of the drug, to bring the level back again.
SINGLE HERBS: Catnip, Chaparral, Hops, Licorice, Lobelia, Skullcap, Slippery Elm, and Valerian.
VITAMINS AND MINERALS: All.
AMINO ACIDS: L-Cysteine, L-Cystine, and L- Methionine.
ALSO: Fasting: drink juice only.

REFERENCES:
"How to Get Well"—P.Airola
"Vitamin Bible"—E. Mindell
"Good News for Smokers"Donsbach

SPASTIC COLON . . . .
Refer to "Colitis" Page 18

STRESS . . . .
HERBAL COMBINATIONS:
(Calm aid) (Ex stress) (Kalmin extract)
PHYSIOLOGIC ACTION: Special formulas for insomnia and stress related conditions. Relieve nervous tension, rebuilds nerve sheaths. Soothing and calming effect on the whole nervous system.
SINGLE HERBS: Black Cohosh Root, Cayenne, Lady's Slipper, Skullcap, and Valerian Root.
VITAMINS: A, all B's, C, D, E, Paba, Folic Acid, & Choline.
MINERALS: Calcium, Chromium, Copper, Iron, Selenium, and Zinc.
ALSO: L-Tyrosine and Protein.
REFERENCES:
"Stress"—Donsbach
"The Athletes Bible" — Global
"The Fitness Formula" — S. Sokol

STRETCH MARKS . . .
Refer to "Skin Problems" P.44

STROKE . . . . .
HERBAL COMBINATION:
(Garlicin HC)
PHYSIOLOGIC ACTION: A combination of herbs which supports the cardiovascular system. Helps to strengthen the heart, while building and cleansing the arteries and veins.
SINGLE HERBS: Cayenne, Comfrey, Evening Primrose Oil, Fish Oil, Garlic, Golden Seal, and Rose Hips.
VITAMINS: B Complex, C, E, Niacin, Inositol, and Choline.

MINERALS: A Multi-mineral, plus Calcium, and Magnesium.
ALSO: Cold pressed vegetable oils..
REFERENCES:
"Natural Treatments & Remedies"
"The Complete Natural Health Encyclopedia"—D. Nyholt

SUNBURN . . . . .
Refer to "Skin Problems" P. 44

TEETH AND GUMS . .
(Toothache)
SINGLE HERBS: Chamomile, Echinacea, Lobelia, Myrrh Gum, and White Oak Bark.
VITAMINS: A, B complex, C, D, P, Folic Acid.
MINERALS: Calcium, Magnesium, Phosphorus, and Silicon.
ALSO: Protein and Unsaturated Fatty Acids.
1. Toothache — Primrose oil or oil of cloves.
2. Stained or yellow teeth — brush with fresh strawberries.
REFERENCES:
"Nutrition Almanac"J. Kirschmann
"Herbally Yours"—P. Royal
"How to Get Well"—P. Airola

TEETH GRINDING . .
SINGLE HERBS: Chamomile, and Skullcap.
VITAMINS: Multi vit., B complex. Take tablets before bed for best results.
ALSO: Bonemeal or other Calcium supplement.
REFERENCES:
"How to Get Well"—P. Airola
"Vitamin Bible"—E. Mindell

TEETHING . . . . .
SINGLE HERBS: Lobelia Extract, Aloe Vera Gel, or Peppermint Oil can be rubbed on the gums.
TISSUE SALTS: combination "R."

ALSO: Teething Tablets from Hylands.
REFERENCES:
"Herbally Yours"—P. Royal

TENSION . . . . .
Refer to "Stress" Page 45

THYROID . . . . .
HERBAL COMBINATION: (T.)
PHYSIOLOGIC ACTION: Rich in natural vitamins and minerals, this excellent formula helps revitalize and promote healing of the thyroid glands thus restoring metabolism balance. Helps the body store up needed vitality and energy.
SINGLE HERBS: Black Walnut, Irish Moss, Kelp, Mullein, and Parsley.
VITAMINS: B1, B5, C, D, E, F.
MINERALS: Chlorine, Iodine, Potassium, and Zinc.
ALSO: Thyroid glandular
REFERENCES:
"Herbally Yours"—P. Royal
"Health Through God's Pharmacy"—M. Treben

TINNITUS . . . . .
HERBAL COMBINATION: (H Formula) (Ginkgold)
PHYSIOLOGIC ACTION: Improves circulation and pulse rate, giving a warming and calming sensation to the ears.
SINGLE HERBS: Cayenne, Black Cohosh, Bayberry, Butchers Broom, Ginkgo, and Yarrow.
VITAMINS: A, B Complex, B3, B6, C, and E.
MINERALS: Calcium, Magnesium, Manganese, and Potassium.
ALSO: Bio-Strath, Coenzyme Q10, and Lecithin.
REFERENCES:
"Nutrition Almanac"J. Kirschmann
"Global Herb Manual"Z. Fortesvn

"Natural Treatments & Remedies"—Global Health
"The Complete Natural Health Encyclopedia"—D. Nyholt

TIREDNESS .....
Refer to "Fatigue General" Page 24

TONSILITIS .....
HERBAL COMBINATIONS: (IF) (IGL)
PHYSIOLOGIC ACTION: Effective formulas that helps cleanse toxins, combat infections, and reduce infection. Especially effective for healing lymphatic system.
SINGLE HERBS: Bayberry Root, Echina Guard, Echinacea, Ginger Root, and Pau d' Arco.
VITAMINS AND MINERALS: A complete one a day multi complex.
ALSO: Canaid herbal drink.

TOOTHACHE .....
Refer to "Teeth and Gums" Page 46

TRENCH MOUTH ....
Refer to "Gingivitis" Page 26

TUMORS (BENIGN) .
SINGLE HERBS: Dandelion, Kelp, Pau d'Arco, and Red Clover.
VITAMINS: A, B5, B6, B Complex, C, and E.
MINERALS: A high potency Multi-mineral.
ALSO: Coenzyme Q10, Germanium, Lecithin, Proteolytic Enzymes, and Sheep Sorrel is an excellent poultice for external tumors.
REFERENCES:
"Nutrition Almanac"—J. Kirschmann
"Natural Treatments & Remedies"—Global Health
"The Complete Natural Health Encyclopedia"—D. Nyholt

ULCERS - (SKIN) ...
HERBAL COMBINATION: (Myrrh – Golden seal)
PHYSIOLOGIC ACTION: Ingredients needed by the body to heal ulcers, cuts, wounds, bruises, sprains and burns. Good as a poultice for external wounds.
VITAMINS: Folic Acid, Panothenic Acid, C, and E.
MINERALS: A Multi-mineral complex.
ALSO: Aloe Vera
Skin ulcers that do not heal — Vitamin E, topical application of comfrey root and/or tea leaf. Dress with a paste made of raw garlic on gauze for 8-10 hours. Take Vitamin C, A, zinc and Calcium orally.
REFERENCES:
"The Aloe Vera Handbook"—M. Skousen
"How to Get Well"—P. Airola

ULCERS - (STOMACH)
HERBAL COMBINATION: (Myrrh – Gold Seal Plus)
SINGLE HERBS: Cayenne (stomach ulcers only), Golden Seal, Myrrh, Pau d'Arco, Red Raspberry, Slippery Elm Bark, Valerian, and White Oak Bark.
VITAMINS: A, B complex, B2, B5, B6, B12, C, D, E, P, Choline, and Folic acid.
MINERALS: Calcium, Manganese, and Zinc,
ALSO: Acidophilus, Chlorophyll, Raw Cabbage, Potato juice, Goat's milk, Brewer's yeast, Aloe Vera, and Halibut oil.
Refer to "Digestive Disorders" in this manual.
REFERENCES:
"The Aloe Vera Handbook"—M. Skousen
"Nutrition Almanac"J. Kirschmann
"How to Get Well"—P. Airola
"Natural Treatments & Remedies"—Global Health

VAGINAL PROBLEMS
(GYNECOLOGICAL PROBLEMS)
HERBAL COMBINATION: (Fem-Mend)
PHYSIOLOGIC ACTION: Menstrual regulator, tonic for genito-urinary system. Helpful for severe menstrual discomforts. Acts as an aid in rebuilding a malfunctioning reproductive system (Uterus, ovaries, fallopian tubes, etc.)
SINGLE HERBS: Aloe Vera, Blessed Thistle, Comfrey Root, Garlic, Ginger, Golden Seal Root, Red Raspberry, Slippery Elm Bark, Uva Ursi, and Yellow Dock Root,
VITAMINS: A, B complex, C, and E.
MINERALS: A Multi-mineral complex.

VAGINITIS . . . . .
HOMEOPATHIC FORMULA: (Vaginitis formula)
PHYSIOLOGIC ACTION: For natural relief of minor vaginal burning and itching.
SINGLE HERBS: Garlic and Pau d'Arco.
VITAMINS: A, B Complex, B6, C, and D.
MINERALS: Calcium and Magnesium.
ALSO: Acidophilus, Protein, and Unsaturated fatty acids.
REFERENCES:
"Natural Treatments & Remedies"
"The Complete Natural Health Encyclopedia"—D. Nyholt

VARICOSE VEINS . . .
PHYSIOLOGIC ACTION: Age, lack of exercise and chronic constipation are contributing factors to varicose veins. B and C vitamins are necessary for the maintenance of strong blood ves-sels. Research has indicated vitamin E improves circulation by dilating blood vessels.
SINGLE HERBS: Butchers Broom, Hawthorn, Horsechestnut, Marigold, Mistletoe, Witch Hazel, White Oak Bark, and Yarrow.
VITAMINS: B complex, C, and E.
MINERALS: Potassium and Zinc.
ALSO: Acidophilus, Protein, and Unsaturated Fatty Acids.
REFERENCES:
"Nutrition Almanac"J. Kirschmann
"Indian Herbology of N America"—A. Hutchens
"Vitamin Bible"—E. Mindell

WARTS - COMMON . .
SPECIFICS: 28000 IU vitamin E oil applied twice a day is an effective treatment.
SINGLE HERBS: Echinacea, Garlic, Golden Seal, and Pau d'Arco.
VITAMINS: — A, B Complex, C, and E(dry form).
MINERALS: Zinc.
REFERENCES:
"Vitamin Bible"—E. Mindel
"How to Get Well"—P. Airola

WATER RETENTION .
HERBAL COMBINATIONS: (KB)
PHYSIOLOGIC ACTION: A mild diuretic to rid the body of excessive water.
SINGLE HERBS: Buchu, Cranberry, Dandelion, Juniper, Parsley, and Uva Ursi.
Note: Limited consumption of common table salt
VITAMINS: B6 and C.
MINERALS: Calcium, and Potassium.
Refer to "Edema" in this manual.
REFERENCES:
"Herbally Yours"—P. Royal
"How to Get Well"—P. Airola
"The Fitness Formula" — S. Sokol
"The Athletes Bible" — Global

"Natural Treatments & Remedies"
"Vitamin Bible"—E. Mindell

WEIGHT CONTROL ..

HERBAL COMBINATIONS:
(SKC) or (Herbal Slim)
PHYSIOLOGIC ACTION: A special, well balanced combination that helps control your appetite, dissolve excess fat, ease stress and anxiety, gently cleanse the bowels, eliminate excess water, and in conjunction with your diet and exercise program, helps you lose weight naturally. Safe and effective.
SINGLE HERBS: Guar Gum, & Konjac Root.
VITAMINS: A, C, and E.
MINERALS: Multi-mineral Complex.
ALSO: Super D's tea, Slim tea, Spirulina diet, Bee Pollen, and Grapefruit Plus.
REFERENCES:
"Lose Weight Feel Great"—J. Yudkin
"All New F Plus Diet"—A Eyeton
"Fit for Life"—H. and M. Diamond
"The Athletes Bible" — Global
"The Fitness Formula" — S. Sokol

WEIGHT GAIN (UNDERWEIGHT) ...

VITAMINS: B complex.
SINGLE HERBS: Bitter herbs such as those found in Swedish Bitters will stimulate appetite.
ALSO: Digestive enzymes, unsaturated fatty acids, and protein.
REFERENCES:
"The Athletes Bible" — Global Health
"The Fitness Formula" — Steve Sokol

WHOOPING COUGH .

HERBAL COMBINATION: (A-P)
PHYSIOLOGIC ACTION: A natural way to ease chronic pain associated with nervous tension, spasms and whooping cough.
SINGLE HERBS: Elecampane, Horehound, Kalmin, Mouse Ear, Sundew, Valerian Root, Wild Cherry Bark, and Wild Lettuce.

WORMS .....

HERBAL COMBINATION:
(Para-X) (Para-VF)
PHYSIOLOGIC ACTION: Para-X is useful in destroying and eliminating parasites. Para-VF is a liquid and is used for children and the elderly who cannot swallow capsules.
SINGLE HERBS: Black Walnut, Garlic, Pumpkin Seeds, and Wormwood.
VITAMINS: Folic Acid.
ALSO: Swedish Bitters.
REFERENCES:
"Nutrition Almanac"J. Kirschmann
"Natural Treatments & Remedies"—Global Health
"The Complete Natural Health Encyclopedia"—D. Nyholt

WRINKLES .....
Refer to "Skin Problems" Page 44

YEAST INFECTION ..

HERBAL COMBINATIONS:
(Garlicin) (Control, caprinex)
PHYSIOLOGIC ACTION: Excellent well balanced formulas for control and eventual elimination of candida overgrowth.
SINGLE HERBS: Black Walnut, Garlic, and Pau d'Arco.
VITAMINS: A, C, E, and Biotin.
ALSO: Primrose oil, Protein, and Primadophilus.
REFERENCES:
"Natural Treatments & Remedies"—Global Health
"Candida Albicans"—L. Chaitow
"The Yeast Connection"—Crook

VITAMINS — NATURAL OR SYNTHETIC ?.....

It is a Global opinion that vitamins in their natural, balanced state are essential for better assimilation, synergistic action and maximum biological effect. As a rule of thumb — if the source is not given the product is synthetic. There are however, a growing number of natural supplement manufacturers that use synthetic vitamins, but use the words natural and/or organic on their labels, in order to mislead the public. The guide below will help you break through the deliberate labeling confusion used by some companies. Don't be misled, be an expert label reader even in a health food store.

Vitamin   *Source Given*

Vitamin		Source Given
Vitamin A	*(Natural)*	*Carrot powder, fish oils, or lemon grass.*
Vitamin A	(Synthetic)	Acetate or palmitate.
Vitamin B1	*(Natural)*	*Rice bran or yeast.*
Vitamin B1	(Synthetic)	Thiamine hydrochloride, thiamine chloride, or thiamine mononitrate.
Vitamin B2	*(Natural)*	*Rice bran or yeast*
Vitamin B2	(Synthetic)	Riboflavin.
Vitamin B3	*(Natural)*	*Rice bran or yeast.*
Vitamin B3	(Synthetic)	If source not given.
Vitamin B5	*(Natural)*	*Yeast.*
Vitamin B5	(Synthetic)	Calcium pantothenate.
Vitamin B9	*(Natural)*	*Yeast.*
Vitamin B9	(Synthetic)	Pteroylglutamic acid.
Vitamin B12	*(Natural)*	*Cobalamine, cyanocobalamin, liver or yeast.*
Vitamin B13	*(Natural)*	*Calcium orotate, or orotic acid.*
Vitamin B15	*(Natural)*	*Calcium pangamate.*
Vitamin B17	*(Natural)*	*Apricot, peach or plum pits.*
B Complex	*(Natural)*	*Brewer's yeast, or soy beans.*
B Complex	(Synthetic)	Choline bitartrate, or d-biotin.
Vitamin C	*(Natural)*	*Rose hips, acerola, or citrus fruits.*
Vitamin C	(Synthetic)	Ascorbic acid or source not given.
Vitamin D	*(Natural)*	*Fish oils.*
Vitamin D	(Synthetic)	Calciferol, or irradiated ergosterol.
Vitamin E	*(Natural)*	*D-alpha tocopherol, tocopherol acetate, mixed tocopherols, wheat germ or veg. oils.*
Vitamin E	(Synthetic)	Alpha tocopherol acetate, or dl-alpha. tocopherol, dl-alpha tocopheryl or acetate.
Vitamin F	*(Natural)*	*Linseed oil or vegetable oils.*
Vitamin H	*(Natural)*	*Yeast.*
Vitamin H	(Synthetic)	D-biotin.
Vitamin K	*(Natural)*	*Alfalfa.*
Vitamin K	(Synthetic)	Menadione.
Vitamin P	*(Natural)*	*Citrus bioflavonoids, citrin, hesperidin, or rutin.*
Vitamin T	*(Natural)*	*Sesame seed.*
Vitamin U	*(Natural)*	*Cabbage extract.*

DOSAGES — VITAMINS & MINERALS

Continual debate rages over what is an (adequate) daily intake of vitamins and minerals. The guide below is just that — a guide only. RDA and Margin of Allowances, are based on the needs of an average adult 23 to 50 years of age, with no special health problems.

	US RDA for adult, 23-50**		Margin of Allowance**	
ViITAMINS				
Vitamin A	5,000 IU		5-10 times RDA	
Thiamin (B1)	1.4 mg		200 times RDA	
Riboflavin (B2)	1.6 mg		588 times RDA	
Niacin (B3)	20 mg		50 times RDA	
Pantothenic acid (B5)	10 mg		100 times RDA	
Pyridoxine (B6)	2 mg		900 times RDA	
Folic acid (B9)	4 mcg		1000 times RDA	
Cobalamin (B12)	6 mcg		n/a	
Orotic acid (B13)	n/a		n/a	
Calc. Pangamate (B15)	(50 mg)	***	(100 mg)	****
Laetrile (B17)	n/a		n/a	
Vitamin C	60 mg		33-83 times RDA	
Vitamin D	400 IU		2.5-5 times RDA	
Vitamin E	10 mg		40 times RDA	
Vitamin F	n/a		n/a	
Vitamin (biotin) H	3 mcg		167 times RDA	
Vitamin K	70 mcg	***	(250 mcg)	****
MINERALS				
Calcium	1000 mg		10 times RDA	
Chlorine	500 mg		(1500 mg)	****
Chromium	(50 mcg)	***	n/a	
Cobalt	(6 mcg)	***	n/a	
Copper	2 mg		5.5 times RDA	
Fluorine	(1 mg)	***	(1.5-4 mg)	****
Iodine	150 mcg		13 times RDA	
Iron	10 mg males		5.5 times RDA	
Iron	18 mg females		5.5 times RDA	
Lithium	n/a		n/a	
Magnesium	400 mg		15 times RDA	
Manganese	2.5-5 mg		n/a	
Molybdenum	(150 mcg)	***	(500 mcg)	****
Phosphorus	1000 mg		10 times RDA	
Potassium	2000 to 2500 mg		n/a	
Selenium	(50 mcg)	***	(150 mcg)	****
Silicon	n/a		n/a	
Sodium	200 to 600 mg		(2 grams)	****
Sulphur	n/a		n/a	
Vanadium	n/a		n/a	
Zinc	15 mg		33 times RDA	

*   US (Recommended Daily Allowances) are based on estimates by the National Academy of Sciences/National Research Council.
**   Adapted from John Hathcock's "Quantitative Evaluation of Vitamin Safety," Pharmacy Times, May 1985.
*** Estimate only — from global health research on data available.
**** Usual therapeutic dose.
RDAs and Margin of Allowances courtesy of the "Natural Life Magazine" Burnaby, B.C., Canada

Vitamins

Vitamin	**Natural Sources**	**Affected Components**
A (Fat Soluble) RDA 5000 IU	Fish liver oils, liver, carrots, green leafy vegetables (kale, turnip greens, spinach), Colorado fruits, melon, squash, yams, tomatoes, margarine, eggs, milk and dairy products	Bones, eyes, hair, mucous linings, membranes, nails, skin, and teeth.
B1 Thiamine (Water soluble) RDA 1.4 mg	Brewers yeast, wheat germ, rice polishings, all seeds, nuts and nut butters, soy beans, beets, potatoes, leafy green vegetables, milk and dairy products.	Brain, ears, eyes, hair, heart, nervous system, and muscles.
B2 Riboflavin (Water soluble) RDA 1.6 mg	Milk, liver, kidney, cheese, fish, eggs, whole grains, brewers yeast, torula yeast, wheat germ, almonds, sunflower seeds, cooked leafy vegetables	Eyes, skin, nails, and hair.
B3 Niacin (Water soluble) RDA 20 mg	Liver, lean meat, white meat of poultry, kidney, fish, eggs, roasted peanuts, avocadoes, dates, figs, prunes, green vegetables, whole wheat products, brewers yeast, wheat germ, rice bran, rice polishings, and sunflower seeds.	Brain, gastro-intestinal tract, nervous system, liver, and skin.

Functions	*Deficiency Symptoms*	*Therapeutic Uses*
Visual purple production (necessary for night vision), promotes growth and vitality, resists infection, repairs and maintains body tissue, helps prevent premature aging and senility.	Allergies, appetite loss, blemishes, dry hair, fatigue, itching/burning eyes, loss of smell, night blindness, rough dry skin, sinus trouble, soft tooth enamel, and susceptibility to infections.	Acne, alcoholism, allergies, arthritis, asthma, athletes foot, boils, bronchitis, colds, cystitis, diabetes, carbuncles, eczema, heart disease, peptitis, migraine headaches, hyperthyroidism, psoriasis, sinusitis, stress, tooth and gum disorders.
Appetite, blood building, carbohydrate metabolism, circulation, aids digestion, energy, growth, learning capacity, prevents liquid retention, prevents constipation, and muscle tone maintenance (intestine, stomach, heart).	Appetite loss, beriberi, digestive disturbances, fatigue, irritability, muscular weakness, nervousness, numbness of hands and feet, mental depression, pains around heart, and shortness of breath.	Alcoholism, anemia, congestive heart failure, fluid retention, constipation, diarrhea, diabetes, indigestion, lead poisoning, nausea, mental illness, pain, rapid heart rate, and stress.
Aids growth and reproduction, alleviates eye fatigue, antibody & red blood cell formation, promotes healthy skin, nails and hair metabolism.	bloodshot and burning eyes, cataracts, corner of mouth cracks & sores, dizziness, poor digestion, premature wrinkles, retarded growth, red sore tongue	Arteriosclerosis, baldness, cholesterol (high), cystitis, facial oiliness, hypoglycemia, light sensitivity, mental retardation, muscular disorders, nervous disorders, and nausea in pregnancy.
Circulation, cholesterol level, dilates blood vessels, hydrochloric acid production, metabolism (protein, fat carbohydrate), tones nervous system, and sex hormone production.	Appetite loss, canker sores, cold feet and hands, depression, fatigue, halitosis, headaches, indigestion, insomnia, muscular weakness, nausea, nervous disorders, and pellagra.	Acne, baldness, canker sores, diarrhea, halitosis, high blood pressure, leg cramps, migraine headaches, schizophrenia, poor circulation, stress, and tooth decay.

Vitamins continued

Vitamin	Natural Sources	Affected Components
B5 Pantothenic Acid (Water soluble) RDA 10 mg	Green vegetables, peas and beans, peanuts, crude molasses, liver, egg yolk, royal jelly, brewers yeast, wheat germ, wheat bran, whole grain breads and cereals.	Brain, digestive system, adrenal glands, mercies system, and skin.
B6 Pyridoxine (Water soluble) RDA 2 mg	Brewers yeast, bananas, avocadoes, wheat germ, wheat bran, cantaloupe, milk, eggs, beef, liver, kidney, heart, blackstrap molasses, soybeans, walnuts, peanuts, pecans, green leafy vegetables, green peppers and carrots.	Blood, muscles, nerves, and skin.
B9 Folic Acid (Water soluble) RDA 4 mcg	Brewers yeast, wheat germ, mushrooms, nuts, liver, broccoli, asparagus, lima beans, lettuce, spinach and deep green leafy vegetables.	blood, glands, hair, liver and skin.
B12 Cobalamin (Water soluble) RDA 6 mcg	Comfrey leaves, kelp, bananas, peanuts, concord grapes, sunflower seeds, brewers yeast, wheat germ, bee pollen, liver, beef, eggs, pork, milk, cheese, and kidney.	Red blood cells, nerves, and brain.
B13 Orotic Acid (Calcium orotate) RDA N/A	Root vegetables, whey, the liquid portion of soured or curdled milk.	Cells, and liver.

Functions	*Deficiency Symptoms*	*Therapeutic Uses*
Aids in wound healing, antibody formation, carbohydrate, fat, protein conversion (energy), growth stimulation, and vitamin utilization.	Blood and skin disorders, constipation, diarrhea, duodenal ulcers, eczema, hypoglycemia, intestinal disorders, kidney trouble, loss of hair, muscle cramps, premature aging, respiratory infections, restlessness, nerve problems, and vomiting.	Allergies, asthma, arthritis, baldness, cystitis, digestive disorders, duodenal ulcers, hypoglycemia, tooth decay, and stress.
Alleviates nausea, antibody formation, digestion (hydrochloric acid production), fat and protein utilization (weight-control), and maintains sodium / poassium balance (nerves).	Acne, anemia, arthritis, convulsions in babies, depression, dizziness, nervous disorders, hair loss, irritability, learning disabilities, muscle spasms, urination problems, and weakness.	Alcoholism, allergies, anemia, arthritis, bronchial asthma, bursitis, epilepsy, fatigue, glossitis, hypoglycemia, insomnia, premenstrual edema, neuritis, overweight, shingles, stress, and seborrheic.
Analgesic for pain, appetite, body growth & reproduction, division of body cells, hydrochloric acid production, improves lactation, protein metabolism, and red blood cell formation.	Anemia, canker sores, digestive disturbances, graying hair, growth problems, impaired circulation, fatigue, and mental depression.	Anemia, arteriosclerosis, baldness, cholesterol (high), constipation, heart disease, loss of libido, overweight, and macrocytic anemia
Appetite, blood cell formation, cell longevity, increases energy and memory, nervous system, metabolism, and promotes growth.	Chronic fatigue, general weakness, nervousness, pernicious anemia, poor appetite, walking, and speaking difficulties.	Baldness, brain damage, dermatitis, eczema, leg cramps, and pernicious anemia.
Essential for the biosynthesis of nucleic acid and regenerating cells.	Not known.	Multiple sclerosis.

Vitamins continued

Vitamin	Natural Sources	Affected Components
B15 Calcium Pangamate (Water soluble) RDA N/A	Whole grains, whole brown rice, pumpkin seeds, sesame seeds, nuts, and brewers yeast.	Kidneys, glands, heart, and nerves.
B17 Laetrile Nitrilosides RDA N/A	Whole seeds — apricot, peach and plum pits, mung beans, lima beans, garbanzos, black-berries, blueberries, cranber-ries, raspberries, millet and flaxseed.	Not known.
Biotin B Complex (Water soluble) also Vit-H RDA 3 mcg	Brewers yeast, fruits, nuts, soybeans, unpolished rice, beef, liver, egg yolk, milk, and kidney.	Hair, skin, and muscles.
Choline B complex (Water soluble) RDA N/A	Granular or liquid lecithin, brewers yeast, wheat germ, egg yolk, liver, and green leafy vegetables.	Brain, hair, gallbladder, kidneys, liver, thymus gland, and controls cholesterol buildup.
Inositol B complex (Water soluble) RDA N/A	Liver, brewers yeast, beef brains and heart, cabbage, citrus fruits, cantaloupe, raisins, wheat germ, whole grains, peanuts, lecithin, milk, and unrefined molasses.	Brain, heart, kidneys, liver muscles, hair and skin.

Functions	Deficiency Symptoms	Therapeutic Uses
Aids recovery from fatigue, cell oxidation & respiration, metabolism (protein, fat, sugar), glandular and nervous system stimulation.	Heart disease, nervous and glandular disorders.	Alcoholism, asthma, arteriosclerosis, cholesterol (high), emphysema, heart disease, headaches, hypoxia, insomnia, poor circulation, premature aging, rheumatism, and shortness of breath.
Purported to have cancer controlling and preventive properties.	May lead to diminished resistance to malignancies.	Cancer.
Antiseptic, cell growth, fatty acid production, hair growth, metabolism (carbohydrate, fat, protein), and vitamin B utilization.	Dandruff, depression, dry skin, fatigue, grayish skin, heart abnormalities, color, insomnia, muscular pain, and poor appetite.	Alcoholism, arteriosclerosis, baldness, cholesterol (high), constipation, dizziness, eczema, ear noises, dermatitis, hardening of the arteries, headaches, heart trouble, high blood pressure, hypoglycemia, insomnia, and seborrhea.
Controls cholesterol buildup, lecithin formation, liver and gall bladder regulation, lowers blood pressure, metabolism (fats, cholesterol), nerve transmission	Bleeding stomach ulcers, cirrhosis, growth problems, heart trouble, high blood pressure, impaired liver & kidney function, and intolerance to fats.	Alcoholism, anemia, arteriosclerosis, Alzheimer's disease, baldness, cirrhosis, diarrhea, fatigue, menstrual problems, mental illness, stomach ulcers, and stress.
Artery hardening retardation, calming effect, cholesterol reduction, hair growth, lecithin formation, metabolism (fat and cholesterol), and preventing eczema.	Cholesterol (high), constipation, eczema, eye abnormalities, and hair loss.	Eczema, obesity, schizophrenia baldness, high blood pressure, and poor circulation.

Vitamins continued

Vitamin	*Natural Sources*	*Affected Components*
Paba B complex (Water soluble) RDA N/A	Liver, kidney, molasses, brewers yeast, rice bran, whole grains, wheat germ, green vegetables, peas, beans, peanuts, egg yolk,	Hair, skin, intestines, and thyroid gland.
C Ascorbic acid (Water soluble) RDA 60 mg	Rose hips, citrus fruits, apples, black currants, strawberries, cabbage, broccoli, cauliflower, persimmons, guavas, tomatoes, sweet potatoes, turnip greens, and green bell peppers.	Ligaments, bones, skin, gums, heart, teeth, blood, adrenal glands, and capillary walls.
D Ergosterol (Water soluble) RDA 400 IU	Egg yolks, milk, butter, fish liver oils, sardines, herring, salmon, tuna, sprouted seeds, mushrooms, and sunflower seeds.	Bones, heart, nerves, skin, teeth, and thyroid gland.
E Tocopherol (Fat soluble) RDA 10 mg	Wheat germ, brussel sprouts, leafy greens, whole wheat, whole grain cereals, vegetable oils, soybeans, and eggs.	Blood vessels, heart, liver, lungs, adrenal and pituitary glands, testes, uterus and fatty tissues.

Functions	*Deficiency Symptoms*	*Therapeutic Uses*
Aids in reproductive disorders, blood cell formation, graying hair, (color restoration), intestinal bacteria, activity protein metabolism, and reduces pain from burns.	Anemia, constipation, depression, digestive disorders, fatigue, gray hair, headaches, irritability, and loss of libido.	Anemia, baldness, graying hair, overactive thyroid, gland parasitic diseases, rheumatic fever, stress, infertility. External: burns, dry skin, sunburn, and wrinkles.
Accelerates healing after surgery, bone & tooth formation, collagen production, common cold prevention, digestion, heals wounds, burns, and bleeding gums, iodine conservation, red blood cell formation, shock & infection resistance, and protection against cancer-producing agents.	Anemia, hemorrhages, capillary wall ruptures, bruise easily, dental cavities, low infection resistance (colds), premature aging, poor digestion, soft and bleeding gums, and thyroid insufficiency.	Alcoholism, asthma, arteriosclerosis, arthritis, cholesterol (high), colds, cystitis, hypoglycemia, heart disease, hepatitis, insect bites, pyorrhea, prickly heat, scurvy, sinusitis, stress, and tooth decay.
Aids in assimilating vitamin A, calcium & phosphorus metabolism (bone, teeth, heart action, nervous system maintenance, normal blood clotting, skin respiration.	Diarrhea, insomnia, myopia, muscular weakness, nervousness, premature aging, poor metabolism, softening bones and teeth, tooth decay.	Acne alcoholism, allergies, arthritis, cystitis, pyorrhea, psoriasis, osteomalacia, osteoporosis, and rickets.
Anti-coagulant, alleviates fatigue, dilates blood vessels, blood cholesterol reduction, improves circulation, capillary wall strengthening, fertility, male potency, lung protection (antipollution), muscle and nerve maintenance, prevents and dissolves blood clots.	Anemias, dry, dull or falling hair, enlarged prostrate gland, gastrointestinal disease, heart disease, impotency, premature aging, miscarriages, muscular wasting, sterility, and tooth decay.	Allergies, arteriosclerosis, baldness, blood clots, cholesterol (high), cystiotos, diabetes, menopausal and menstrual disorders, migraine headaches, myopia, phlebitis, sinusitis, stress, sterility, thrombosis, varicose veins. External: burns, scars, warts, and wounds.

Vitamins continued

Vitamin	Natural Sources	Affected Components
F Linoleic & Linolenic (Fat soluble) RDA N/A	Vegetable oils — wheat germ, almonds, avocados, peanuts, sunflower seeds, walnuts, soybeans, safflower and linseed oil.	Adrenal and thyroid glands, cells, hair, nerves, skin, heart and arteries.
H Biotin RDA 3 mcg	Also a B Complex. See Page 56.	
K Menadione (Fat soluble) RDA N/A	Kelp, alfalfa, liver, yogurt, egg yolk, safflower and soybean oil, fish liver oil, and leafy green vegetables.	Blood, and liver.
P Rutin Bioflavonoids (Water soluble) RDA N/A	Apricots, blackberries, cherries, buck wheat and the white skins and segment part of all citrus fruit.	Blood, bones, capillary walls, gums, ligaments, skin, and teeth.
T Sesame Seed Factor	Sesame seeds, sesame butter, and egg yolks.	Blood.
U (Fat soluble) RDA N/A	Raw cabbage juice, fresh cabbage, and sauerkraut.	Stomach.

Functions	Deficiency Symptoms	Therapeutic Uses
Burns, saturated fat, blood coagulation, blood pressure normalizer, cholesterol destroyer, combats heart disease, influences glandular activities, promotes healthy hair and skin, and vital organ respiration.	Acne, allergies, diarrhea, dry skin, dry brittle hair, eczema, falling hair, gall stones, kidney disorders, nail problems, prostrate disorders, underweight, and varicose veins.	Acne, allergies, baldness, bronchial asthma, cholesterol (high), eczema, gall bladder and kidney problems or removal, heart disease, leg ulcers, psoriasis, rheumatoid arthritis, overweight, and underweight.
Activates energy producing tissues, blood clotting (coagulation), and important for normal liver function.	Bleeding ulcers, diarrhea, increased tendency to hemorrhage and miscarriages, lowered vitality, and nose bleeds.	Bruising, eye hemorrhages, celiac disease, colitis, gall stones, hemorrhaging, menstrual problems, preparing women for childbirth, and ulcers.
Aids in healing bleeding gums, blood vessel wall maintenance, bruising minimization, cold & flu prevention, and strong capillary maintenance.	Bleeding gums, cirrhosis of the liver, eczema, hemorrhaging, hardening of arteries, and respiratory infections.	Asthma, bleeding gums, colds, eczema, edema, dizziness, hemorrhoids, high blood pressure, hypertension, miscarriages, rheumatic fever, rheumatism, and ulcers,
Combats anemia hemophilia, improves memory.	Not known	Anemia and hemophilia.
Promotes healing in peptic ulcers.	Not known.	Peptic ulcers and duodenal ulcers.

Minerals

Mineral	Natural Sources	Affected Components
Calcium RDA 800 to 1200 mg	Milk, cheese, sardines, salmon, soybeans, dark leafy vegetables, sesame seeds, oats, navy beans, almonds, millet, walnuts, sunflower seeds, and tortillas.	Bones, teeth, nails, blood, heart, skin, and soft tissue.
Chlorine RDA 500 mg	Kelp. watercress, avocado, chard, cabbage, kale, celery, asparagus, cucumber, olives, tomatoes, turnip, and saltwater fish.	Blood, liver, and stomach.
Chromium RDA N/A	Brewers yeast, cane sugar, meat, shell fish, chicken, clams, and corn oil.	Arteries, and blood.
Cobalt RDA N/A	All green leafy vegetables, clams, kidney, liver, oysters, milk, and red meat.	Blood.
Copper RDA 2 mg	Beef liver, seafood, almonds, beans, peas, prunes, raisins, whole grain products, and green leafy vegetables.	Blood, bones, brain, connective tissues, and nerves.
Fluorine RDA N/A	Milk, cheese, carrots, garlic, sunflower seeds, seafood, and fluoridated drinking water.	Bone, and teeth.
Germanium RDA N/A	Garlic, aloe, comfrey, chorella, ginseng, and water cress.	All cells.
Iodine RDA 150 mcg	Kelp, dulse, seafood's and fish liver oils, egg yolks, citrus fruits, artichokes, garlic, turnip greens, watercress, pineapples, and pears.	Hair, nails, thyroid gland, brain, skin, and teeth.

Functions	*Deficiency Symptoms*	*Therapeutic Uses*
Bone/tooth formation, blood clotting, heart rhythm, nerve tranquilization, nerve transmission, and muscle growth and contraction.	Heart palpitations, insomnia, muscle cramps, nervousness, arm & leg numbness, and tooth decay.	Arthritis, aging symptoms (backache, bone pain, finger tremors, foot/leg cramps, insomnia, menstrual cramps, menopause problems, nervousness, overweight, premenstrual tension, and rheumatism.
Maintains fluid and electrolyte balance, helps liver, and production of hydrochloric acid.	Impaired digestion, loss of hair and teeth, and derangement of fluid levels in the body.	Digestion, stomach acidity, and stiffness of joints.
Blood sugar level, glucose metabolism (energy).	Arteriosclerosis, glucose intolerance in diabetics.	Diabetes, and hypoglycemia.
Aids in hemoglobin formation.	Development of pernicious anemia.	Anemia.
Development of bones, brain, nerves and connective tissues, hair & skin color, healing processes of body, hemoglobin and red blood cell formation.	General weakness, impaired respiration, and skin sores.	Anemia, and baldness.
strengthens bones, reduces tooth decay	not known	tooth decay
A relatively new mineral. builds immune cells, gives energy, and has rejuvenative properties.	Not known.	Anemia.
Energy production, metabolism (excess fat), physical and mental development.	Cold hands and feet, dry hair, irritability, nervousness, and obesity.	Arteriosclerosis, hair problems, goiter, and hyperthyroidism.

Minerals continued

Mineral	Natural Sources	Affected Components
Iron RDA 10 mg. males 18 mg. females	Apricots, peaches, bananas, black molasses, prunes, raisins, whole rye, walnuts, brewers yeast, kelp, dulse, dry beans and lentils, liver, kidney, heart, egg yolks, red meat, oysters, and raw clams.	Blood, bones, nails, skin, and teeth.
Lithium RDA N/A	Kelp, dulse, and seafood.	Nerves, muscles, and brain.
Magnesium RDA 350 mg	Apples, figs, lemons, peaches, kale, endive, chard, celery, alfalfa, beet tops, whole grains, brown rice, sesame seeds, sunflower seeds, almonds, and yellow corn.	Arteries, bones, heart, muscles, nerves, and teeth.
Manganese RDA N/A	Nuts and grains, spinach, beets, Brussels sprouts, peas, kelp, wheat germ, apricots, blueberries, egg yolks, and citrus fruits.	Brain, thyroid and mammary glands, muscles, and nerves.
Molybdenum RDA N/A	Brown rice, millet, buck wheat, legumes, leafy vegetables, brewers yeast, and whole cereals.	Blood.
Phosphorus RDA 800 to 1200 mg	Dairy products, whole grains, seeds and nuts, egg, fish, poultry, meat, dried fruits, legumes and corn.	Bones, brain, heart, kidneys, nerves, and teeth.

Functions	Deficiency Symptoms	Therapeutic Uses
Hemoglobin production, stress and disease resistance.	Breathing difficulties, brittle nails, iron deficiency, anemia (pale skin, fatigue), and constipation.	Alcoholism, anemia, colitis, and menstrual problems.
Helps transport sodium metabolism to brain nerves and muscles.	Nervous and mental disorders.	Paranoid schizophrenic.
Acid and alkaline balance, blood sugar metabolism (energy), and metabolism (calcium & vitamin C).	Confusion, disorientation, easily aroused anger, nervousness, rapid pulse, and tremors.	Alcoholism, cholesterol (high), depression, heart conditions, kidney stones, nervousness, prostrate troubles, sensitivity to noise, stomach acidity, tooth decay, overweight.
Enzyme activation, reproduction & growth, sex hormone production, tissue respiration, vitamin B1 metabolism, and vitamin E utilization.	Ataxia (muscle coordination failure), dizziness, ear noises, and loss of hearing.	Allergies, asthma, diabetes, and fatigue.
Integral part of enzymes involved in oxidation processes.	Unknown.	Copper poisoning and improper carbohydrate metabolism
Bone/tooth formation, cell growth & repair, energy production, heart muscle contraction, kidney function, metabolism (calcium, sugar), nerve & muscle activity, and vitamin utilization.	Appetite loss, fatigue, irregular breathing, nervous disorders, overweight, and weight loss.	Arthritis, stunted growth in children, stress, and tooth and gum disorders.

Minerals continued

Mineral	Natural Sources	Affected Components
Potassium RDA 2000 to 2500 mg	All vegetables, bananas, citrus fruits, cantaloupe, tomatoes, water cress, sunflower seeds, whole grains, potatoes, milk, and mint leaves.	Blood, heart, kidneys, muscles, nerves, and skin.
Selenium RDA N/A	Wheat germ, brewers yeast, kelp, garlic, mushrooms, onions, tomatoes, broccoli, seafood's, milk, eggs, and bran.	Blood, prostrate gland, liver, and testicles.
Silicon RDA N/A	Flaxseed, steel cut oats, almonds, peanuts, sunflower seeds, apples, strawberries, grapes, kelp, beets, onions, and parsnips.	Bones, hair, nails, and teeth.
Sodium RDA 200 to 600 mg	Sea salt, kelp, shellfish, carrots, celery, asparagus, romaine lettuce, beets, dried beef, brains, kidney, bacon and watermelon.	Blood, lymph system, stomach, muscles, and nerves.
Sulfur RDA N/A	Radish, turnip, onions, celery, horseradish, kale, soybeans, water cress, eggs, fish, and lean beef.	Hair, skin, nails, and nerves.
Vanadium RDA N/A	Fish.	Heart and blood vessels.
Zinc RDA 15 mg	Sprouted seeds, wheat bran and germ, pumpkin seeds, sunflower seeds, brewers yeast, onions, nuts, green leafy vegetables, lean beef, lamb chops, pork loin, eggs, oysters, and herring.	Blood, brain, heart, and prostrate gland.

Functions	**Deficiency Symptoms**	**Therapeutic Uses**
Heartbeat, rapid growth, muscle contraction, and nerve tranquilization.	Acne, continuous thirst, dry skin, constipation, general weakness, insomnia, muscle damage, nervousness, slow irregular heartbeat, and weak reflexes.	Acne, alcoholism, allergies, burns, colic in infants, diabetes, high blood pressure, and heart disease (angina pectoris, congestive heart failure, myocardial infraction).
Antioxidant, slows aging process and hardening of tissues through oxidation.	Premature stamina loss.	Degenerated liver, impotence, and mercury poisoning.
Building of strong bones, helps healing process and builds immune system, normal growth of hair, nails and teeth.	Aging symptoms of skin (wrinkles), thinning or loss of hair, poor bone development, and soft or brittle nails.	Hair loss, irritations in mucous membranes, skin disorders, and insomni.a.
Helps nerves and muscles function properly and normalizes glandular secretions.	Excessive sweating, chronic diarrhea, nausea, respiratory failure, heat exhaustion, and impaired carbohydrate digestion.	Sun stroke, heat prostration, muscular weakness, and mental apathy.
Collagen synthesis and body tissue formation.	Not known.	Arthritis. External: skin disorders (eczema, dermatitis, psoriasis).
Inhibits formation of cholesterol in blood vessels.	High blood pressure and hardening of arteries.	Aids in preventing heart attacks, and high blood pressure.
Burn and wound healing, carbohydrate digestion, prostrate gland function, reproductive organ growth and development, sex organ growth and maturity.	Delayed sexual maturity, fatigue, loss of taste, poor appetite, prolonged wound healing, retarded growth, and sterility.	Alcoholism, arteriosclerosis, baldness, cirrhosis, diabetes, internal & external wound & injury healing, high cholesterol (eliminates deposits), and infertility.

A WORD ABOUT HERBS

SINGLE HERBS
A herb with medical properties used by Herbalists for the prevention and correction of disease. All herbs in this book are presented for the express purpose of making it easy for the layman to use.

HERBAL COMBINATIONS
Herbal combinations consist of two or more herbs selected and compounded to cover symptoms of specific diseases. A single herb often does not have all of the therapeutic qualities that are required.

HERBAL SYRUPS AND TINCTURES
When immediate results are needed, the liquid extracts are suitable because of their rapid absorption. They can be added to small amounts of juice, water, and herb teas to make them more palatable.

HERBAL DOSAGES
You should only use the dosages recommended by the manufacturer as the strengths can vary. The quantities and frequencies written on the labels are for adults weighing approximately 150 lbs. When using herbal remedies for children or the elderly, the use should be decreased. Herbal capsules may be prepared as a tea. To make sure that the herbs are properly assimilated, they should be taken with a full glass of water.

SINGLE HERBS

ALFALFA
Medicinal Parts: Flowers, Leaves, Petals, and Sprouts.
Actions and Uses: Very high in vitamin and minerals thus nourishes the entire system. Excellent for pregnant women and nursing mothers. Good for the pituitary gland. It alkalizes the body rapidly and helps detoxify the liver. Helps rebuild decayed teeth and relieve arthritic and rheumatic pain. Also aids in the assimilation of protein, fats and carbohydrates. Contains an anti fungus agent.
Bodily Influence: Nutrient, Tonic.

ALFA-MAX
Medicinal Part: Leaves.
Actions and Uses: A concentrated alfalfa extract made from the leaves of alfalfa, Alfalfa surpasses all other natural, unprocessed foods in vitamin and mineral content. Approximately one ton of green alfalfa makes 80 lbs. of Alfa-Max.
Bodily Influence: Nutrient, Tonic.

ALOE VERA
Medicinal Part: Leaves.
Actions and Uses: Aloe Vera is a potent medicine and healer. An excellent colon cleanser. Healing and soothing to the stomach as well as liver, kidneys, spleen and bladder. Also an excellent remedy for piles and hemorrhoids. Works

Single Herbs (continued)

with your immune system to keep you healthy, strong and vibrant.
Bodily Influence: Anthelmintic, Emmena- gogue, Purgative, and Tonic.

ANGELICA

Medicinal Parts: Herb, Root and Seed.
Actions and Uses: Resists poisons, aids in expulsion of gas from the stomach and intestines, also good for colic, grip and heartburn. Promotes secretion of fluid from respiratory track. Tea taken hot will quickly break up a cold.
Bodily Influence: Aromatic, Carminative, Diaphoretic, Diuretic, Emmenagogue, Expectorant, and Stimulant.

ASTRAGLUS

Medicinal Part: Root.
Actions and Uses: Strengthens the immune systems and promotes healing. It strengthens resistance to disease and improves digestion.
Bodily Influence: Anhydrotic, Diuretic, and Tonic.

BARBERRY

Medicinal Parts: Bark, Berries and Root.
Actions and Uses: and blood tonic.
External use — antiseptic root tea. Also used for kidney ailments.
Bodily Influence: Antiseptic, Laxative, Stimulant, and Tonic.

BARLEY GRASS

Medicinal Part: Leaves.
Actions and Uses: Excellent source of chlorophyll, used to treat rheumatic and arthritic symptoms. Barley water gives relief in fevers, diarrhea and stomach irritations.

Bodily Influence: Demulcent, and Nutritive.

BAYBERRY

Medicinal Part: The root bark.
Actions and Uses: Astringent and stimulant effective in cleaning congestion from the nose and sinuses. Good for all mucus membrane conditions. Made into a tea it is excellent as a gargle for sore throats. Valuable for all kinds of hemorrhages.
Bodily Influence: Astringent, Stimulant, and Tonic.

BEE POLLEN

Medicinal Part: Fresh pollen from bees.
Actions and Uses: A miracle food from nature rich in vitamins, minerals and amino acids. Reduces the craving for protein. Used for aging, prostrate gland, fatigue, allergies and as a sexual rejuvenate. Also contains natural antibodies so is effective against infections.
Bodily Influence: Antimicrobial and Antiseptic.
Warning: Some people may be allergic to bee pollen. Use small amounts at first and discontinue if discomfort or any other symptoms occur.

BEET POWDER

Medicinal Part: Root.
Actions and Uses: One of the best-known plant sources of assumilable iron. Good for toning and rebuilding liver also gall bladder infections. Also contains Vitamin A, B, C, sodium, potassium, calcium and chlorine.
Bodily Influence: Adaptogen, Hepetic, and Nutritive.

Single Herbs (continued)

BILBERRY

Medicinal Part: Leaves and Berries.

Actions and Uses: Bilberry has a well established reputation as being similar to insulin for sugar diabetes. Useful for diarrhea, dropsy, gravel, liver and stomach conditions.

Bodily Influence: Astringent, Diuretic, and Refrigerant.

BLACK COHOSH

Medicinal Part: Root.

Actions and Uses: A natural precursor to estrogen; helps relieve symptoms such as premenstrual and menstrual cramps. Lowers cholesterol and high blood pressure (equalizes circulation), helpful for poisonous bites, reduces mucus levels, and relieves sinusitis and asthma.

Bodily Influence: Alterative, Anti-spasmodic, Cardiac Stimulant, Diuretic, Diaphoretic, Emmenagogue, Expectorant, and Sedative (arterial and nervous)

Warning: Do not take if you are pregnant or have any type of chronic disease.

BLACK WALNUT

Medicinal Parts: Bark, Husks, Leaves, Rind, and Green Nut.

Actions and Uses: Expels internal parasites and tape worms. Should be applied topically to ring worm twice a day until it disappears. Aids in treatment of tuberculosis, diarrhea, and promotes healing of sores in mouth and throat. Rich in manganese which is important for nerves, brain and cartilage, and helps relieve many kinds of skin problems.

Bodily Influence: Tonic, and Vermifuge.

BLADDERWRACK

Medicinal Parts: Leaves and Root.

Actions and Uses: Eliminates parasites, improves goiter and kidney functions, increases thyroid activity, and absorbs water in the intestines to produce bulk.

Bodily Influence: Adaptogen, and Vermifuge.

BLESSED THISTLE

Medicinal Parts: Flower, Leaves, Root, and Seed.

Actions and Uses: Stimulates appetite, promotes menstrual discharge, helps regulate hormones, increase milk production while nursing, also a stimulant to brain, circulation, heart and nerves.

Bodily Influence: Adaptogen, Galact-agogue, and Stimulant.

Warning: Handle carefully to avoid toxic skin effects.

BLUE COHOSH

Medicinal Part: Root.

Actions and Uses: Relieves or prevents spasms, cramps, colic, diabetes, leukorrhea, nervous disorders, rheumatism. Elevates blood pressure, cleanses blood, promotes perspiration also increases volume of urine excreted.

Bodily Influence: Antispasmodic, Depurative, Diuretic, Dysmenorrhea, Emmenagogue, Oxytocic, Parturient, Sudorific and Spasmodic.

BLUE VERVAIN

Medicinal Parts: Leaves, Root, and Stems.

Actions and Uses: Expels worms, increases and restores proper

Single Herbs (continued)

blood circulation, relieves bladder, helps to expel phlegm from the throat and lungs. Good for asthma, epilepsy, colds, female disorders, fever, flu, headaches, and pneumonia.

Bodily Influence: Antiperiodic, Anti-pasmodic, Diaphoretic, Emetic, Expectorant, Nervine, Sudorific, and Tonic.

BONESET

Medicinal Parts: Leaves and Tops.

Actions and Uses: Mild laxative, reduces fevers, promotes perspiration. Also used in the treatment of acute and chronic rheumatism.

Bodily Influence: Antispasmodic, Aperient, Diaphoretic, Emetic, Stimulant, and Tonic.

BUCHU

Medicinal Part: Leaves.

Actions and Uses: Used for chronic inflammation of the bladder, digestive disorders, irritation of the urethra, urine retention, nephritis, cystitis and catarrh of the bladder.

Bodily Influence: Antiseptic, diuretic, and stimulant,

BURDOCK

Medicinal Parts: Leaves, Seed, Stems, Root, (the whole herb).

Actions and Uses: Cleanses and eliminates impurities from the blood, thus alleviating boils, abscesses, eczema and other skin disorders. An excellent diuretic. Soothing to the kidneys. Excellent for gout and will reduce arthritic swelling, deposits within the joints.

Bodily Influence: Alterative, Diaphoretic, and Diuretic.

Warning: Burdock interferes with iron absorption.

BUTCHER'S BROOM

Medicinal Parts: Seeds, and Tops.

Actions and Uses: Builds up structure of the veins. Therefore used for hemorrhoids and other types of varicose veins. Improves poor circulation, also relieves inflammation in the kidney and bladder.

Bodily Influence: Demulcent, Mucilaginous, Rubifacient, and Styptic.

CDN. SNAKE ROOT

Medicinal Part: Root.

Actions and Uses: Accelerates childbirth causing stimulation of the involuntary muscles of the uterus. Relieves gas from stomach and intestines. Promotes perspiration and increases volume of urine excreted.

Bodily Influence: Carminative, Parturient, and Stomachic.

CAPSICUM (CAYENNE)

Medicinal Part: The fruit.

Actions and Uses: A catalyst for all herbs. Capsicum taken with Burdock, Ginger, Golden Seal, Slippery elm, etc., will soon diffuse itself throughout the whole system. Improves circulation, and aids digestion. Combine with Lobelia for nerves. Unlike most stimulants of allopathy, it is not narcotic. Good for the heart, lungs kidneys, pancreas, spleen, and stomach.

Bodily Influence: Carminative, Condiment, Diaphoretic, Rubefacient, Stimulant, and Tonic.

Single Herbs (continued)

CASCARA SAGRADA

Medicinal Part: Dried Bark.
Actions and Uses: One of the best natural laxatives in the herbal kingdom. Extremely useful in hemorrhoidal conditions and chronic constipation. It is considered suitable for delicate and elderly persons. Also a very good remedy for gallstones, increases secretion of bile.
Bodily Influence: Laxative, and Bitter tonic.

CATNIP

Medicinal Parts: The whole herb.
Actions and Uses: Excellent for small children with colic. Controls fever (catnip enemas reduce fever) Produces perspiration without increasing body temperature. Very good as a sleeping aid, relieves stress and is soothing to the nerves. Also a digestive aid for gas and diarrhea.
Bodily Influence: Antispasmodic, Aphrodisiac (cats), Carminative, Diaphoretic, Emmen-agogue, Stimulant, and Tonic.

CELERY

Medicinal Parts: Root and Seed.
Actions and Uses: Used in incontinence of dropsical, urine, and liver problems. Good for arthritis, rheumatism, neuralgia, and nervousness. Acts as an antioxidant and a sedative.
Bodily Influence: Aromatic, Carminative, Diuretic, Nerve Sedative, Stimulant, and Tonic.

CHAMOMILE

Medicinal Parts: Flowers and Herb.
Actions and Uses: A natural sedative for hysteria, nightmares, delirium and nervousness also used as a digestive aid for weak stomachs and to provide appetite.
Bodily Influence: Antispasmodic, Carmin-ative, Diaphoretic, Emmenagogue, Nervine, Sedative, and Tonic stimulant.
Warning: Do not use for long periods of time. Do not use if allergic to ragweed.

CHAPARRAL

Medicinal Parts: Leaves and Stem.
Actions and Uses: Blood purifier. One of natures best antibiotics very useful in cases of acne, arthritis, chronic backache, tumor warts and skin blotches. Protects from harmful effects of radiation and sun exposure, also used for liver problems, lymphatic troubles and digestive disorders.
Bodily Influence: Antiseptic, Diuretic, Expectorant, and Tonic.

CHICKWEED

Medicinal Parts: Whole Herb.
Actions and Uses: Used extensively to help lose weight. Excellent herb for the digestive system and bowels. One of the best remedies for tumors piles and swollen testes. Excellent bronchial cleanser. Heals and soothes.
Bodily Influences: Demulcent, Emollient, Pectoral, and Refrigerant.

CHLORELLA

Medicinal Parts: Fresh spear leaves. (barley or wheat)
Actions and Uses: Highest known source of natural chlorophyll stimulates the natural immune system. Also very effective in

Single Herbs (continued)

detoxifying the liver, bloodstream and in cleansing the bowel. Chlorella helps clear heavy metals and harmful chemicals from the body.
Bodily Influences: Alterative, Depurative, Hepatic, Nutritive, and Stimulant.

CLEAVERS

Medicinal Part: Whole Herb.
Actions and Uses: Acts as a solvent of stones in the bladder. Helps with urinary secretion. Also used for treatment of scurvy, psoriasis, skin diseases and eruption generally.
Bodily Influences: Alterative, Aperient, Diuretic, Refrigerant, and Tonic.

CODONOPSIS

Medicinal Part: Root.
Actions and Uses: Called "poor mans ginseng" in China. Has very similar qualities as ginseng, and can be used by both sexes in any climate.
Bodily Influences: Adaptogen and Tonic.

COLTSFOOT

Medicinal Parts: Berries and Leaves.
Actions and Uses: For congestion of the pulmonary system, especially if inclined to consumption. Also used for asthma, bronchitis, coughs, catarrh, diarrhea, fever, inflammation, and ulcers.
Bodily Influence: Demulcent, Emollient, Expectorant, Pectoral, and Tonic.
Warning: Carcinogenic properties have been discovered.

COMFREY

Medicinal Parts: Leaves and Root.
Actions and Uses: Good blood cleanser and tissue builder, help to heal broken bones, sprains and slow healing sores. Helps heal ulcers and kidney problems. Best remedy for blood in urine. Also a powerful remedy for coughs and catarrh.
Bodily Influence: Astringent, Demulcent. *Warning:* Do not use for longer than 3 months at a time. May cause liver damage.

CORNSILK

Medicinal Part: The green pistils.
Actions and Uses: Corn Silk will assist all inflammatory conditions of the bladder, kidney, and urethra. Controls general malfunction of the body due to uric acid retention. Good for hypertension, edema, urinary tract dysfunction, and stones, bedwetting, and enlarged prostrate gland.
Bodily Influence: Alterative, Demulcent, and Diuretic.

CRANBERRY

Medicinal Part: Fruit.
Actions and Uses: Good for chronic kidney infections also used for relief of cramps and spasms of involuntary muscular contractions such as in asthma and hysteria.
Bodily Influence: Diuretic, Mucilaginous, and Nervine.

DAMIANA

Medicinal Part: Leaves.
Actions and Uses: A great sexual rejuvenator. Gives energy, helps to balance female hormones.

Single Herbs (continued)

Controls bed wetting, expels excess water from the body. Stimulates muscular contractions of the intestinal tract and increases blood circulation.
Bodily Influence: Aphrodisiac, Laxative, Stimulant, and Tonic.
Warning: Damiana interferes with iron absorption when taken internally.

DANDELION
Medicinal Part: Root.
Actions and Uses: Strengthens kidneys and bladder. Removes excess fluids, gallstones, jaundice and poisons. Excellent for anemia because is high in iron, calcium and other vitamins and minerals. A very good diuretic.
Bodily Influence: Aperient, Deobstruent, Diuretic, Stomachic, and Tonic.

DEVILS CLAW
Medicinal Part: Leaves.
Actions and Uses: A blood cleanser which will remove deposits in the joints and aid in the elimination of uric acid from the body. Very effective for arthritis, gout and rheumatism, as well as liver and kidney disorders.
Bodily Influence: Adaptogen, Alterative, Antirheumatic, and Depurative

DONG QUAI
Medicinal part: Root.
Actions and Uses: Used To treat various female gynecological problems menopause, PMS, and hot flashes. It is the female equivalent of Korean ginseng. Also relieves constipation by moistening the intestinal tract.
Bodily Influence: Adaptogen, Laxiative, and Nutritive.

Warning: Should not be used during pregnancy.

ECHINACEA
Medicinal Parts: Leaves, Dried Rhizome, and Root.
Actions and Uses: Glandular balancer, especially lymphatic and liver areas. Also blood purifier, antiseptic and anti-infection herb. Good for boils, blood poisoning, carbuncles, all pus diseases, snake and spider bites. Helps boost immune response.
Bodily Influence: Alterative, Diaphoretic, and Sialagogue.
Warning: Alcohol tincture may destroy polysaccharides in echinacea that stimulate the immune system.

EVENING PRIMROSE
Medicinal Parts: Bark, Leaves, and Seeds.
Actions and Uses: An excellent source of essential fatty acids (EFA's). Good for skin disorders female disorders such as cramps, hot flashes, heavy bleeding, especially effective against atopic diseases such as eczema, PMS and hyperactivity.
Bodily Influence: Astringent, Nervine, and Sedative

EYEBRIGHT
Medicinal Part: Leaves.
Actions and Uses: It is the main herb for protecting and maintaining the health of the eye. Acts as an internal medicine for the constitutional tendency to eye weakness. Will remove cysts that have been caused by chronic conjunctivitis.
Bodily Influence: Adaptogen, Nutritive.

Single Herbs (continued)

FENNEL

Medicinal Part: Whole Herb.
Actions and Uses: Helps suppress the appetite. Aids digestion when uric acid is the problem. Good for gas, acid stomach, kidneys, liver, spleen, gout and mixed with catnip in tincture form as an aid to colic in infants. Also relieves pain for cancer patients after chemotherapy and radiation.
Bodily Influence: Antispasmodic, Carmin-ative, and Galactagogue.

FENUGREEK

Medicinal Part: Seeds.
Actions and Uses: Useful for all mucus conditions of the lungs. Good for bronchitis, fevers, sore throats and inflammation of stomach and intestines. Also acts as a bulk laxative.
Bodily Influence: Demulcent, Emollient, Expectorant, and Laxative.

FEVERFEW

Medicinal Parts: Whole Herb.
Actions and Uses: Helpful in the prevention of migraines, relieves dizziness, brain and nerve pressure. Stimulates uterine contractions, promotes menses, increases fluidity of lung and bronchial tube mucus. Also used in alleviating inflammation and discomfort of arthritis and female disorders.
Bodily Influence: Aperient, Carminative, Emmenagogue, Stimulant, Tonic, and Vermifuge.

FO-TI

Medicinal Part: Root.
Actions and Uses: Stimulant, excellent for mental depression. Has been used to help the mem-ory. Recent scientific studies verify cholesterol-lowering effects of this herb. Also helps to rejuvenate the endocrine glands which in turn, strengthen the body.
Bodily Influence: Stimulant and Tonic.

GARLIC

Medicinal Part: Bulb.
Actions and Uses: Natural antibiotic, stimulates activity of the digestive organs,. It is used to emulsify the cholesterol and loosen it from the arterial walls. Proven useful in asthma and whooping cough. Valuable in intestinal infections and effective in reducing high blood pressure.
Bodily Influence: Alterative, Antibiotic, and Esculent.

GENTAIN

Medicinal Parts: Leaves and Root.
Actions and Uses: Most useful in states of exhaustion from chronic disease, and all cases of general debility, weakness of digestive organs and want of appetite. Kills plasmodia (organisms that cause malaris) and Worms. Many dyspeptic complaints are effectively relieved with gentian.
Bodily Influence: Adaptogen, Fubrifuge, Nutritive, Stimulant, Tonic, and Vermifuge.

GINKGO

Medicinal Part: Leaves.
Actions and Uses: Widens blood vessels, increases circulation and speeds blood flow in the capillaries. Useful for hearing, vision, senility, dizziness, ringing in ears, heart and kidney disorders.

Single Herbs (continued)

Bodily Influence: Cardiac, Rubifacient, and Vasodilator.

GINGER

Medicinal Part: Root and rhizomes.

Actions and Uses: Hot as tea promotes cleansing of the body through perspiration and useful for suppressed menstruation. Relieves indigestion, gas, morning sickness, nausea. In a recent university study, ginger root capsules proved to be far more effective at controlling motion-induced nausea than either a drug or placebo. It helps absorb toxins, restore gastric activities to normal, and helps control diarrhea and vomiting that often accompanies gastro-intestinal flu.

Bodily Influence: Carminative, Diaphoretic, Diuretic, Stimulant, and Tonic.

GINSENG (KOREAN)

Medicinal Part: Root.

Actions and Uses: A physical restorative. Helps the entire body adapt to stress, regenerates and rebuilds sexual centers. Impotency and low sperm count have been corrected by using Korean Ginseng. Stimulates the appetite, and normalizes blood pressure. Anciently known as a male hormone, and used for longevity.

Bodily Influence: Aphrodisiac, Demulcent, Nervine, Stimulant, and Stomachic.

GINSENG (SIBERIAN)

Medicinal Part: Root.

Actions and Uses: Main action is a tonic and toner of the body, promotes mental and physical vigor, stamina, endurance, metabolism, appetite and digestion. Mildly stimulates the central nervous system, also helpful in problems arising in menopause such as hot flashes and irregular periods. Also good for cocaine withdrawal, radiation protection, and enhances lung, and immune functions.

Bodily Influence: Aphrodisiac, Demulcent, Nervine, Stimulant, and Stomachic.

Caution: Avoid if hyperactive or under high nervous tension.

GOLDEN SEAL HERB

Medicinal Part: Rhizomes.

Actions and Uses: For all problems of the mucus membranes. Contains many of the same properties as the root but in milder form. Relieves nausea. The infusion makes a good vaginal douche.

Bodily Influence: Alterative, Antibiotix, Antiseptic, Emmenagogue, Stomachic, Tonic.

Warning: Do not use large amounts during pregnancy. When used over a long period, will reduce vitamin B absorption.

GOLDEN SEAL ROOT

Medicinal Part: Root.

Actions and Uses: A natural antibiotic herb used with all infections. A powerful agent used in treating ulcers, diphtheria, tonsillitis and spinal meningitis. Combined with Gota Kola, Goldenseal acts as a brain tonic. One of the best substitutes for quinine.

Bodily Influence: Alterative, Antibiotic, Antiseptic, Laxative, and Tonic.

GOTU KOLA

Medicinal Parts: Nuts, Root, and Seeds.

Single Herbs (continued)

Actions and Uses: Known in India as the longevity herb. Contains remarkable rejuvenating properties. May promote hair growth when combined with eclipta. It strengthens the heart, and liver functions. Good for mental disorders, blood diseases, high blood pressure, sore throat, tonsillitis, hepatitis, measles, rheumatism, and venereal diseases. Used as a brain cell activator to help memory.
Bodily Influence: Antibiotic, Nervine, Rubifacient, and Tonic.

GUAR GUM

Medicinal Part: Leaves And Seed.
Actions and Uses: Used as a diet aid because it absorbs liquids and swells, also reduces serum cholesterol levels and has a mild bulk-forming laxative effect.
Bodily Influence: Esculent, and Laxative.

HAWTHORN

Medicinal Part: Berries and Leaves.
Actions and Uses: A dietary herb, aids in burning off excess calories. Relieves abdominal distention and diarrhea. A herbal aid for circulation and specific nutritional resources for building heart tone. Valuable in angina pectoris or inflammation of the heart muscle.
Bodily Influences: Adaptogen, Cardiac, and Circulatory Tonic.

HOPS

Medicinal Parts: Strobiles or Cones.
Actions and Uses: A powerful sedative, strong yet safe to use. Decreases the desire for alcohol, improves appetite and induces sleep. Good for heart, stomach and liver problems, nervousness, restlessness, pain, toothaches, earaches, and stress.
Bodily Influence: Anodyne, Anthelmintic, Diuretic, Febrifuge, Hypnotic, Nervine, Sedative and Tonic.

HOREHOUND

Medicinal Parts: Whole Herb.
Actions and Uses: Used for congestion of coughs, colds, and pulmonary affections associated with unwanted phlegm from the chest. Good for intestinal gas, when taken in large doses it is a laxative and will expel worms.
Bodily Influence: Anthelmintec, Diuretic, Diaphoretic, Expectorant, Laxative, Resolvent, Stimulant, Stomachic, and Tonic.

HORSETAIL (SHAVEGRASS)

Medicinal Parts: Leaves and Stems.
Actions and Uses: Contains a great deal of silica. Increases calcium absorption, promotes healthy skin, strengthens bone, hair, nails, and teeth. Also a diuretic. Helps with kidney disorders, especially kidney stones. Used as poultice to depress bleeding and accelerate healing of wounds.
Bodily Influence: Astringent, Diuretic, Lithotriptic, and Tonic.

HUCKLEBERRY

Medicinal Parts: Whole Plant.
Actions and Uses: Used to lower insulin, blood sugar levels, and to ease inflammation. Good for diabetes, kidney, bladder, sinusitis, and ulcers.

Single Herbs (continued)

Bodily Influences: Alterative, Depurative, Nutritive, and Stomachic. Caution: Interferes with iron absorption when taken internally.

IRISH MOSS

Medicinal Parts: Whole Plant.
Actions and Uses: Used in cosmetics to soften and promote elasticity of the skin. Also effective in the treatment of thyroid problems (goiter), colon disorders, and obesity.
Bodily Influences: Adaptogen, and Emollient.

JUNIPER BERRY

Medicinal Part: Ripe dry berries.
Actions and Uses: Useful in digestive problems, gastrointestinal infections, inflammations, cramps, dropsy kidney, and bladder diseases. Also good for gout, and other arthritic conditions associated with acid waste.
Bodily Influence: Carminative, Diuretic, and Stimulant.
Warning: Not intended for use during pregnancy.

KAVA KAVA

Medicinal Part: Root.
Actions and Uses: An excellent herb for insomnia and nervousness. Invokes sleep and relaxes the nervous system.
Bodily Influence: Antiseptic, Anti-spasmodic, and Diuretic.
Warning: Long term usage of high dosages can interfere with elimination of toxins from the liver.

KELP (NORWEGIAN)

Medicinal Part: Leaves

Actions and Uses: Source of olkaki, calcium, sulphur, iodine, silicon and vitamin k. Beneficial to reproductive organs and tones the walls of the blood vessels. Excellent for the thyroid gland and goiters. Has a remedial and normalizing action on the sensory nerves. Good for nails, hair, and radiation poisoning.
Bodily Influence: Demulcent, Thyroid restorative, and Nutritive.

LADY SLIPPER ROOT

Medicinal Part: Root.
Actions and Uses: Acts as a tonic to the exhausted nervous system, improving circulation and nutrition of the nerve centers. This in turn calms nerves, mental irritation and quiets spasms of voluntary muscles with no harmful or narcotic effects.
Bodily Influence: Antiperiodic, Nervine, and Tonic.

LICORICE ROOT

Medicinal Part: The dried root.
Actions and Uses: Hormone balancer. Natural cortisone. Used for hypoglycemia, adrenal glands, stress, female problems (menstrual and menopause). Muscle or skeletal spasms, and increases fluidity of mucus from the lungs and bronchial tubes. Used for coughs, chest complaints, gastric ulcers, and throat conditions.
Bodily Influence: Demulcent, Expectorant, Laxative, and Pectoral.
Warning: Large doses of licorice root should be avoided by people with high blood pressure.

LOBELIA

Medicinal Parts: Leaves, Flower, Seeds and Stem.

Single Herbs (continued)

Actions and Uses: A powerful relaxant used extensively for persons wishing to stop smoking or drinking. Aids in Hormone production. Reduces palpitation of the heart and strengthens muscle action. Good for fevers, pneumonia, meningitis, pleurisy, hepatitis and peritonitis. The Indians used Red Lobelia for syphilis and for expelling or destroying intestinal worms. Emetic in large amounts.

Bodily Influence: Antispasmodic, Diaphoretic, Emetic, Expectouant, Nauseant, Relaxant, Sedative, and Stimulant.

MARSHMALLOW

Medicinal Parts: Whole Herb.

Actions and Uses: Useful in inflammation and irritation of the alimentary canal, urinary and respiratory organs. Also used in combination with other diuretic herbs during kidney treatment to assist in release of stones.

Bodily Influence: Demulcent, and Emollient.

MILK THISTLE

Medicinal Parts: Fruit, Leaves and Seeds.

Actions and Uses: Regenerates liver cells and protects them against the action of liver poisons (leukotrienes). Beneficial to those with psoriasis. Aids rehabilitation process after acute hepatitis, gall bladder disease or exposure to alcohol, drug or chemical pollution

Bodily Influence: Cholagogue, Liver Tonic.

MILKWEED

Medicinal Part: Root.

Actions and Uses: Used for inflammatory rheumatism, dyspepsia and scrofulous conditions of the blood. A helpful remedy for bowel, kidney, and stomach complaints. Good for female complaints, asthma, arthritis, and bronchitis. Remedy for gall-stones and used for dropsy as it increases the flow of urine.

Bodily Influence: Diaphoretic, and Expectorant.

Warning: May be harmful to children and people over 55.

MULLEIN

Medicinal Parts: Leaves and Flowers.

Actions and Uses: Pain reliever, glandular rebuilder. The only herb known that is a narcotic without being harmful or poisonous. Good for coughs, colds, hay fever, shortness of breath and hemorrhages in lungs. Also used as a treatment for hemorrhoids.

Bodily Influence: Anodyne, Antispasmodic, Astringent, Demulcent, Diuretic, and Pectoral.

MYRRH GUM

Medicinal Part: Leaves.

Actions and Uses: Stimulator, appetite and flow of gastric juices. A powerful antiseptic which is generally used in equal parts with golden seal for intestinal ulcer, catarrh of the intestines and other mucus membrane conditions. Also used for bronchial and lung diseases. Tightening the gums and preventing pyorrhea is one of its most outstanding qualities.

Bodily Influence: Antiseptic, Digestive Aid, and Stimulant.

NETTLE

Medicinal Parts: Roots and Leaves.

Single Herbs (continued)

Actions and Uses: Tradition use, asthma relief, also used for kidney diseases, colon and urinary disorders, checking hemorrhage of uterus, nose, lungs and other internal organs. Nettle is valuable in diarrhea, dysentery, piles, neuralgia, gravel, and tea made from the young or dried root is of great help in dropsy of the first stages.

Bodily Influence: Astringent, Diuretic, Pectoral, and Tonic.

External Use: Cleansing wounds and ulcers.

OAT BRAN

Medicinal Part: Seed.

Actions and Uses. Contains soluble and insoluble fiber, which have cholesterol-lowering benefits. Also useful in maintaining a healthy colon.

Bodily Influence: Adaptogen and Esculent.

OREGON GRAPE

Medicinal Part: Fruit.

Actions and Uses: Blood purifier and liver activator. Builder of the reproductive organs. Increases the power of digestion and aids assimilation. Recommended as an alternative for treatment of psoriasis, syphilis and unpure blood conditions. Combine with Cascara Sagrada for constipation.

Bodily Influence: Alterative, Esculent, and Tonic.

PARSLEY

Medicinal Parts: Leaves, Seeds, and Root.

Actions and Uses: Rich in vitamin B and potassium. An excellent diuretic, and one of the most excellent herbs for gall bladder problems. Expels gallstones. Also good for bed wetting, edema, fluid retention, goiter, gas, indigestion, menstrual disorders, and worms. Also useful as a preventative in treating Epilepsy.

Bodily Influence: Anthelmintic, Aperient, Carminative, Diuretic, Esculent, Expectorant and Stimulant.

Caution: Shouldn't be used if the kidney is inflamed. Avoid heavy consumption during pregnancy.

PASSION FLOWER

Medicinal Parts: Plant and Flower.

Actions and Uses: When in need of help for nervousness, unrest, agitation and exhaustion without pain, such as unrest, agitation, and exhaustion, Passion Flower is helpful. Also used to control convulsions, particularly in the young, as indicated by muscular twitching, and also for asthenic insomnia in childhood and the elderly;

Bodily Influence: Anodyne, Antispasmodic, Diuretic, and Nerve Sedative.

PAU D'ARCO

Medicinal Parts: Inner Bark.

Actions and Uses: Undoutably the greatest treasure the Incas left us. Medical literature confirms that this South American herb possesses antibiotic, tumor inhibiting, virus killing, anti fungal, and anti-malarial properties. Consumer publications report success for the symptoms of anemia, asthma, candida, psoriasis, colitis, and resistance to various infections by building the immune system. Due to genetic mutation resistant strains of candida develop rapidly. Patients who no longer respond to Pau d'Arco will

Single Herbs (continued)

find that rotating treatment with Mathake tea to be beneficial.
Bodily influence: Adaptogen, Antibiotic, Nutritive, and Resolvent.

PENNYROYAL

Medicinal Parts: Whole Plant:
Actions and Uses: Diuretic, corrective nervine used to induce perspiration and promote menstruation. Purifies the blood, stimulates uterine contractions, relieves gas and intestinal pains. Also for nervousness and hysteria, cramps, gout, colic, jaundice, nausea, griping, colds. and skin disorders.
Bodily Influence: Corrective, Diaphoretic, Diuretic, and Nervine.
Warning: Do not use during pregnancy.

PEPPERMINT

Medicinal Parts: Flowers and Leaves:
Actions and Uses: Irritates the gastrointestinal tract, mucous membranes, and increases stomach acidity. Used to relieve gas pains, nausea, dysentery, diarrhea and stop vomiting. Also good for chills, colic, fevers, dizziness, influenza and palpitation of the heart.
Bodily Influence: Adaptogen, Antacid, Carminative, cariac, and Pectoral.
Warning: May interfere with Iron absorption.

PLANTAIN

Medicinal Parts: Whole Plant:
Actions and Uses: Influences lymphatic system and builds tissue. Excellent remedy for kidney and bladder problems. Also used externally on inflamed skin with malignant ulcers, external hemorrhaging, insect bites, burns, scalds and ulcers.
Bodily Influence: Alterative, Antiseptic, Astringent, and Diuretic.

PROPOLIS

Bees manufacture propolis to prevent disease from entering the hive. As it is a natural antibiotic it wards off all kinds of infections such as colds, flu, fevers, digestive disorders, etc.

PSYLLIUM

Medicinal Part: Seed.
Actions and Uses: Psyllium assists in easy evacuation by increasing water in the colon, cleans out compacted pockets thereby making bowel movements easier for people with colitis and hemorrhoids. Creates bulk. Relieves auto-intoxication.
Bodily Influence: Demulcent, and Laxative.
Warning: Because Psyllium forms an indigestible mass, it should be taken at different times than other supplements.

PUMPKIN

Medicinal Part: Seed and Husks.
Actions and Uses: Used for worms, stomach problems, morning sickness, nausea, and toning the prostate gland.
Bodily Influence: Adaptogen, Anthelmintic, Nervine, and Vermifuge.

QUEEN OF MEADOW

Medicinal Part: Root.
Actions and Uses: One of the best known herbs for kidney and bladder infections. Valuable in diarrhea, especially for children.

Single Herbs (continued)

Imparts to the bowels some nourishment as well as an astringency.
Bodily Influences: Antacid, Carminative, Demulcent, and Diuretic.

RED CLOVER

Medicinal Part: Blossoms, and Leaves..
Actions and Uses: An excellent blood purifier, glandular restorer and mineralize. Contains silica and other earthy salts. Good for tuberculoses and to fight other bacteria, inflamed lungs, whooping cough, gout, and arthritis. Relaxing to nerves and entire system. Also used for many years as an antidote to cancer.
Bodily Influence: Adapogen, Alterative, Antibiotic, Discutient, Nutritive, Sedative, and Tonic.

RED RASPBERRY

Medicinal Parts: Whole plant.
Actions and Uses: Effective in menstrual problems, decreasing the blood flow without stopping it abruptly. Promotes healthy nails, bones, teeth, and skin. Remedy for dysentery and diarrhea in infants. Tea excellent for morning sickness in pregnancy. Helps prevent miscarriage, and strengthens uterine walls prior to giving birth. Long-term usage may be required to achieve optimal results.
Bodily Influence: Astringent, Stimulant, and Tonic.
Warning: May interfere with iron absorption.

RESHI MUSHROOM

Medicinal Part: Top.
Actions and Uses: Has a positive effect on the immune system. Good for allergies and auto- immune diseases. Acts as an immune modulator. Has a reported anti- tumor activity. Aids the liver and is helpful for digestion. Has antibacterial and anti viral properties. It has been used for bronchitis, coronary disease, senility and general debility. Used in recent years to treat patients suffering with AIDS.
Bodily Influence: Adaptogen, Alterative, Demulcent, Dicsutient, Esculent, Nutritive, and Tonic.

RHUBARB

Medicinal Part: Root.
Actions and Uses: Useful for colon, spleen, and liver disorders. Enhances gallbladder functions and has a positive effect on duodenal ulcers. Good for headaches, constipation, diarrhea, and hemorrhoids.
Bodily Influence: Adaptogen, Antibiotic, Hepatic, and Stomachic

ROSEHIPS

Medicinal Part: Seed and Pod.
Actions and Uses: An extremely high source of Vitamin C. Thus effective with colds, diarrhea, coughs, consumption, dysentery and scurvy. Also helps to combat stress.
Bodily Influence: Adaptogen, Antiseptic, and Nervine.

SAFFRON

Medicinal Part: Leaves and Root.
Actions and Uses: A natural hydrochloric acid (utilizes sugar of fruits/oils), thus helping arthritics get rid of the uric acid which holds the calcium deposited in joints. Also reduces lactic acid build up.
Bodily Influence: Antacid, Antirheumatic.

SAGE

Medicinal Part: leaves.

Single Herbs (continued)

Actions and Uses: Best known effect is the reduction of perspiration and stopping the flow of milk in a nursing mother. Also used for nervous conditions, trembling, depression and vertigo.
Bodily Influence: Astringent, Diaphoretic, Expectorant, and Tonic.

SANICLE - SNAKEROOT

Medicinal Parts: Root and Leaves.
Actions and Uses: Possesses powerful cleansing and healing properties both internally and externally. Good for asthma, boils, debility diabetes, diarrhea, gastritis, dysentery, intermittent fevers, lungs, intestines, ozaena, reproductive organs, renal tract, and throat discomfort.
Bodily Influence: Alterative, Anodyne, Astringent, Discutient, Nervine, and Vulnerary.

SARSAPARILLA

Medicinal Part: Root.
Actions and Uses: Widely used by athletes as a natural steroid and as a source of precursors of muscle building hormones. Clears skin disorders such as eczema, and psoriasis. Increases energy, and protects against harmful radiation. Eliminates poisons from the blood and helps cleanse the system of infections. Useful for rheumatism, gout, skin eruptions, ringworm, scrofula, internal inflammation, colds and catarrh.
Bodily Influence: Alterative, Antiscoubutic, Demulcent, Diuretic, and Stimulant.

SAW PALMETTO

Medicinal Part: Berries.

Actions and Uses: A tissue builder. It is recommended in all wasting diseases as it has a marked effect upon all the glandular tissue. Capable of increasing nutrition of the testicles and mamma in functional atony of these organs. Also builds stamina and endurance and rids respiratory membranes of mucus. Also of use in renal conditions and diabetes.
Bodily Influence: Anti-catarrhal, Diuretic, Expectorant, Nutritive, Sedative, and Tonic

SCHIZANDRA FRUIT

Medicinal Part: Root.
Actions and Uses: Used to enhance the immune system. Has an a positive effect on the lungs. Used in some cases for forgetfulness. Also used for insomnia.
Bodily Influence: Adaptogen, Anti-catarrhal, Nervine, and Sedative.

SCULLCAP

Medicinal Part: Whole Herb.
Actions and Uses: A natural antidepressant. More effective than quinine, and not harmful. Good for neuralgia, aches and pains, rheumatism, convulsions, and nervous tension. Helps reduce high blood pressure, helps heart conditions and disorders of the central nervous systems such as palsy, hydrophobia and epilepsy.
Bodily Influence: Antispasmodec, Nervine, Relaxant, and Restorative.

SENNA

Medicinal Part: Leaves.
Actions and Uses: A stimulant laxative, extremely powerful,

Single Herbs (continued)

should be combined with ginger or fennel to prevent cramping. Will help eliminate most types of worms from the colon if used following wormwood. Use externally for skin diseases and pimples.

Bodily Influence: Cathartic, Laxative, and Vermifuge.

Warning: Do not use during pregnancy or if there is inflammation in intestinal tract.

SHEPHERD PURSE

Medicinal Part: Whole Plant.

Actions and Uses: Controls hemorrhaging of stomach, lungs, uterus and kidneys. Also successfully used in cases of hemorrhaging after childbirth and excessive menstruation. Also valuable when used for dysentery, vulnerary, rheumatism, catarrh, dropsy, and chronic menorrhagia.

External Use: Juice stops external bleeding and heals bruises.

Bodily Influence: Antiscorbutic, Astringent, and Diuretic.

SHITAKI MUSHROOM

Medicinal Part: Top.

Actions and Uses: Used as both food and healing agent in the Orient. Taken to enhance the immune system. Has an anti-tumor activity and helps to enhance the natural protective defenses of the body. Will lower blood cholesterol levels and help to pull fat from the system. May be helpful for those diagnosed with clinical depression.

Bodily Influence: Adaptogen, Discutient, Esculent, Stimulant.

SLIPPERY ELM

Medicinal Part: Inner Bark (fresh or dried).

Actions and Uses: Considered one of the most valuable remedies in herbal practice, having wonderful strengthening and healing qualities. Has a soothing and healing action on all parts it comes in contact with. Used extensively for inflammation of the lungs, bowels, stomach, heart, diseases of female organs, kidney and bladder. Slippery Elm will soothe ulcerated or cancerous stomach when nothing else will.

Bodily Influence: Demulcent, Emollient, and Nutritive.

SOLOMON'S SEAL

Medicinal Part: Rhizome.

Actions and Uses: Helps to mend broken bones. Also pulmonary consumption and bleeding of the lungs, female complaints, bruises, hemorrhoids, inflammations of the stomach, and tumors.

Bodily Influence: Astringent, Demulcent, and Tonic.

ST. JOHN'S WORT

Medicinal Parts: Tops and Flowers.

Actions and Uses: This is one of the most useful of herbs, can be used by young or elderly. Useful in stopping bed wetting. Also for treatment of dysentery, diarrhea, bleeding of the lungs, worms, jaundice and suppressed urine. Will also correct irregular menstruation.

Bodily Influence: Astringent, Diuretic, Expectorant, Sedative.

STRAWBERRY

Medicinal Part: Leaves, Root and Berries.

Actions and Uses: A good blood purifier, clears eczema and other skin conditions. Very effective in treating intestinal malfunctions (diarrhea, dysentery and weakness of intestines and urinary organs).

Single Herbs (continued)

Bodily Influence: Mild Astringent, and Diuretic

SQUAW VINE

Medicinal Part: Root.
Actions and Uses: Particularly good for women in building of female organs. It has been used for years by expectant mothers six weeks prior to delivery to aid parturition. Alleviates painful menstruation and is a diuretic. Used for insomnia and also used successfully for gravel and urinary ailments.
Bodily Influence: Adaptogen and Nutritive.

SUMA

Medicinal Parts: Bark, Berries, Leaves, and Roots.
Actions and Uses: Also called Brazilian Ginseng. It is the richest source of naturally-occurring germanium and an immune system booster. It has a positive tonic effect on the endocrine system and helps the body to regulate hormone levels. As a female hormone balancer, Suma will act as a precursor to the production of estrogen if the body needs it. It will not cause the production of more estrogen then the body can handle. Useful for anemia, diabetes, and stress.
Bodily Influences: Adaptogen, and Tonic.

TEA TREE

Medicinal Part: Leaves.
Actions and Uses: Extremely effective as a germicide and fungicide, the antiseptic power of the Tea Tree Oil is 12 times that of carbolic acid. Good for athletes foot, cold sores, cystitis, dermatitis, wounds, and yeast infections.
Bodily Influence: Antiseptic.

THYME

Medicinal Parts: Whole Plant.
Actions and Uses: Used for hysteria, nervous disorders, fever, headaches, and mucus. Lowers cholesterol levels and is good for sinusitis, asthma, and chronic respiratory problems.
Bodily Influence: Antispasmodic, Carmin-ative, Emmenagogue, and Tonic.

UVA URSI

Medicinal Parts: Leaves.
Actions and Uses: Very useful in diabetes and all kinds of kidney and bladder infections. Helps disorders of the small intestines, spleen, liver, and pancreas. Strengthens heart muscle, and imparts tone to the urinary passages. Excellent remedy for piles, hemorrhoids, kidney stones, and helpful in the treatment of gonorrhea. Also good where there are mucus discharges from the bladder with pus and blood.
Bodily Influence: Adaptogen, Anti-syphilitic, Cardiac, Hemostatic, Stimulant, and Tonic.

VALERIAN ROOT

Medicinal Parts: Root, Rhizomes
Actions and Uses: A strong nervine without a narcotic effect. Soothes and quiets the nervous system, beneficial in cardiac palpitation. Used for epileptic fits, nervous tension or irritations. Excellent for children with measles and scarlet fever.
Bodily Influence: Antispasmodic, Calm-ative, Nervine, Stimulant, and Tonic.

Single Herbs (continued)

VIOLET

Medicinal Parts: Leaves and Flowers.

Actions and Uses: Useful for pain in cancerous growths. Soothing and healing effect on inflamed mucal surfaces. Good for colds, hoarseness, inflammation of the lungs, and whooping cough.

Externally: Compress on inflamed tumors, sore throat, and swollen breasts.

Bodily Influence: Antiseptic, and Expectorant.

WATER CRESS

Medicinal Parts: Flower, Leaves, and Root.

Actions and Uses: Helps the body to use oxygen, stimulates rate of metabolism, increasing physical endurance and stamina and improves heart response. Used for Bladder, kidney, and liver problems, and dissolves kidney stones.

Bodily Influence: Alterative, Nutritive, Stimulant, and Tonic.

WHITE OAK BARK

Medicinal Parts: Bark and Acorn.

Actions and Uses: Good for varicose veins. Used in douches and enemas, for internal tumors and swellings. Excellent remedy for, hemorrhoids, hemorrhages, varicose veins, tumors, womb troubles, goiter or any trouble of the rectum. Normalizes the liver, kidneys, spleen, and dissolves kidney stones and gallstones.

Bodily Influence: Antiseptic, Astringent Haemostatic, and Tonic.

WHITE WILLOW BARK

Medicinal Part: Bark.

Actions and Uses: It is one of nature's greatest gifts to mankind as a pain-relieving, fever-lowering, anti-inflammatory agent without any side effects. Helps relieve symptoms of headache, fever, arthritis, rheumatism, bursitis, dandruff, eye problems (eyewash), influenza, chills, eczema and nosebleed. Most effective in concentrated extract form.

Bodily Influence: Anodyne, and Astringent.

WILD YAM- DIOSCOREA

Medicinal Part: Root.

Actions and Uses: Yam is a source of the male sex hormone testosterone and is used for rejuvenating effects. Relieves nauseous symptoms of pregnancy, and will help to prevent miscarriage when combined with ginger. Good for Acne, Angina, Biliousness, Diarrhoea, Dysentery Gall-bladder and Liver disorders.

Bodily Influence: Antispasmodic, Anti-bilious, and Diaphoretic.

WINTERGREEN

Medicinal Part: Whole Plant.

Actions and Uses: Used for centuries for its ability to relieve pains of rheumatism. Also good for headaches, colic, flatulence, gastritis, Neuralgia, pleurodynia, and urinary ailments.

Bodily Influence: Anodyne, Astringent, and Stimulant.

WITCH HAZEL

Medicinal Parts: Bark and Leaves.

Actions and Uses: One of the best known herbs to check internal bleeding, especially for excessive menstruation, hemorrhages from the lungs, stomach, uterus and bowels. Also useful in

Single Herbs (continued)

reducing pain associated to diarrhea, dysentery and hemorrhoids.
Bodily Influence: Astringent, Sedative, and Tonic.

WOOD BETONY

Medicinal Part: Leaves.
Actions and Uses: Strengthens and stimulates the heart muscle. Expels worms. Good for headache, colic, colds, gout, indigestion, and stomach cramps. Also used for jaundice, Parkinson's disease, and tuberculosis.
Bodily Influence: Anodyne, Antacid, Nutri-tive, Stomachic, and Vermifuge.

WORM WOOD

Medicinal Parts: Tops and Leaves.
Actions and Uses: Used for aminorrhoes, chronic leucorrhoea, diabetes, diarrhea, female complaints, inflammation of tonsils and quinsy. Also small doses are used for dispersing the yellow bile of jaundice from the skin caused by liver conditions.
Bodily Influence: Anthelmintix, Febuefuge, Narcotic, Stimulant, Stomachic, and Tonic.
Warning: Overdose will irritate the stomach and increase heart action.

YARROW

Medicinal Parts: Whole Herb.
Actions and Uses: Very high in tannic acid thus helps to stop bleeding wounds, hemorrhaging stomach, bowels and lungs. Also useful in menstrual irregularities and has a soothing effect on nervous conditions of the heart.
Bodily Influence: Alterative, Astringent, Diuretic, and Tonic.

Warning: Interferes with the absorption of iron.

YELLOW DOCK

Medicinal Parts: Leaves and Roots.
Actions and Uses: It is a powerful restorer of the lymphatic system. Also a blood purifier, laxative, astringent and effective in skin problems such as psoriasis, eczema, and urticarea. When made into an ointment it is valuable to use for swelling, open sores and itching eruptions. Combine with Sarsaparilla as a tea for chronic skin disorders.
Bodily Influence: Alterative, Antiscorbutic, Astringent, Laxative, and Tonic.

YERBAMATE

Medicinal Parts: Whole Herb.
Actions and Uses: Used to enhance the healing powers of other herbs. Stimulates the mind, and nervous system, retards aging, and stimulates the production of cortisone. Also good for allergies, hay fever, arthritis, fluid retention, and constipation.
Bodily Influences: Adaptogen, Alterative, Anodyne, Antirheumatic, Nervine, and Sedative.

YUCCA

Medicinal Part: Root.
Actions and Uses: New hope for arthritics. Contains special steroid saponins which are effective in treating acute forms of arthritis and rheumatism. Tests at the University of Wyoming show that Yucca may also have an anti-cancer potential.
Bodily Influence: Alterative, Anti-rheumatic, and Disculient.

Homeopathic Singular Tissue Salts
Amino Acid Supplements

L-Arginine

Metabolizes body fat and tones muscle tissue, increases sperm count in males, aids in the healing of wounds.

L-Aspartic acid

Improves stamina and endurance, increases resistance to fatigue, helps protect the central nervous system.

L-Carnitine

Body fat stores by converting nutrients into energy, enhances athletic performance, disperses excess calories.

L-Cystine

Helps to detoxify the system, aid in protection from smoke, alcohol and heavy metals, also helps protect the body against x-rays and nuclear radiation.

L-Glutamine

Used primarily as a brain fuel (improves intelligence). Alleviates fatigue, and depression, also used in the control of alcoholism.

L-Glycine

Used in the treatment of gastric hyperacidity, academia, low pituitary gland function and progressive muscular dystrophy.

L-Lysine

Improves concentration and mental alertness. Utilizes fatty acids required in energy production, useful in the control and prevention of herpes simplex infection.

L-Methionine

Used in the treatment of edema and some cases of schizophrenia, research indicates a possible link to atherosclerosis and cholesterol deposits.

L-Ornithine

Involved in the release of human growth hormone, converts fat into energy and muscle, strengthens immune system, accelerates tissue repair and wound healing.

L-Phenylalanine

Controls hunger, improves memory, and alertness, enhances sexual interest, helps alleviate depression.

DL-Phenylalanine

A non addictive and non toxic natural pain killer, also is a very strong anti-depressant.

L-Tryptophan

Anti-depressant, reduces anxiety, tension and promotes sleep. Lowers pain sensitivity, also aids in the control of alcoholism.

L-Tyrosine

Appetite depressant, fights fatigue and depression, helps cocaine addicts kick the habit — alleviates the withdrawal symptoms.

A Word About Tissue Salts

Dr. W. H. Schuessler isolated them in the late nineteenth century. Also known as (Schuessler biochemical cell salts). Tissue salts are inorganic mineral components of your body tissues. Dr. Schuessler found that illness occurred if the body was deficient in any of these salts and the body could heal itself if the deficiency was corrected. We recommend that you use only the dosages prescribed on the manufacturer's label as there is a variant in strengths between different manufacturers.

Homeopathic Singular Tissue Salts

Mineral	*Actions & Uses*	*Affected Components*
#1 CALC-FLUOR (Calcium Fluoride) (Fluoride of Lime)	Maintains elasticity of tissues.	Impaired circulation, piles, varicose veins, muscle tendon strain, deficient enamel teeth, carbuncles, cracked skin, and over-relaxed conditions.
#2 CALC-PHOS (Calcium Phosphate) (Phosphate of Lime)	Constituent of bones, teeth, and gastric juices.	Impaired digestion, anemia, cold hands and feet, numbness, hydrocele, teething, sore breasts, and night sweats.
#3 CALC-SULPH (Calcium Sulfate) (Sulfate of Lime)	Blood purifier, constituent of all connective tissue in minute particles.	Acne, skin eruptions, abscesses, pimples during adolescence, sore lips, and chronic oozing ulcers.
#4 FERR-PHOS (Iron Phosphate)	The biochemic first aid oxygenates the blood.	Diarrhea, nosebleeds, coughs, colds, chills, fevers, inflammation, congestion, rheumatic pain, and excessive menses.
#5 KALI-MUR (Potassium Chloride) (Chloride of Potash)	Blood constituent and conditioner. Found in lining under surface body cells.	Coughs, colds, respiratory ailments. also granulation of eyelids, warts, and blistering eczema.

Homeopathic Singular Tissue Salts

Mineral	*Actions & Uses*	*Affected Components*
#6 KALI-PHOS (Potassium Phosphate)	Nerve Nutrient. Found in all nerve, brain, and blood cells.	Nervous exhaustion, indigestion, headaches, poor memory, anxiety, insomnia, and improper fat digestion.
#7 KALI-SULPH (Potassium Sulfate) (Sulfate of Potash)	Oxygenates the tissue salts. Constituent 0f skin cells, and internal organ linings.	Pains in limbs, feeling of heaviness, skin eruptions with sealing or sticky exudation, falling hair, and diseased nails.
#8 MAG-PHOS (Magnesium Phosphate) (Phosphate of magnesia)	Nerve stabilizer and anti-spasmodic. Constituent of bones, teeth, brain, nerves, blood, and muscle cells.	Cramps, neuralgia, shooting pains, flatulence, and colic.
#9 NAT-MUR (Sodium Chloride) (Chloride of Soda)	Water-distribution. Regulates the amount of moisture in the body.	Loss of smell or taste, salt cravings, colds, watery discharges from eyes, and nose.
#10 NAT-PHOS (Sodium Phosphate) (Phosphate of Soda)	Acid-neutralizer. Emulsifies fatty acids and keeps uric acid soluble in the blood.	Over acidity of the blood, jaundice, gastric disorders, heartburn, and rheumatic tendency.
#11 NAT-SULPH (Sodium Sulphate) (Sulphate of Soda)	Excess water eliminator. An irritant to tissues and functions as a stimulant for natural secretions.	liver symptoms, gall bladder disorders, edema, depression, low fevers, bilious attacks, and watery infiltration's.
#12 SILICA (Silicic Oxide) (Silicic Acid)	Conditioner, cleanser, eliminator. Constituent of all connective tissue cells.	Lack of luster or falling hair, boils, impure blood, brittle, ribbed or ingrown nails, carbuncles, and poor memory.

Homeopathic Combination Tissue Salts

Combination	Ingredients	Therapeutic Use
A	Ferr Phos, Kali Phos, Mag Phos	Used for neuritis, neuralgia, and sciatica.
B	Calc Phos, Kali Phos, Ferr Phos	Used during convalescence and general debility.
C	Mag Phos, Nat Phos, Nat Sulph, Silica	For acidity, heartburn, and dyspepsia.
D	Kali Mur, Kali Sulph, Calc Sulph, Silica	Acne, eczema, scalp eruptions, and skin ailments.
E	Calc Phos, Mag Phos, Nat Phos, Nat Sulph	For flatulence, colic and indigestion.
F	Kali Phos, Mag Phos, Nat Mur, Silica	For nervous headaches, migraine when associated with nervous weakness.
G	Calc Fluor, Calc Phos, Kali Phos, Nat Mur	For backache, lumbago, piles, and overrelaxed condition of the tissues.
H	Mag Phos, Nat Mur, Silica	Hay fever.
I	Ferr Phos, Kali Sulph, Mag Phos	Fibrosis and muscular pains
J	Ferr Phos, Kali Mur, Nat Mur	A seasonal remedy for coughs and colds.
K	Kali Sulph, Nat Mur, Silica	Falling hair, brittle nails.
L	Calc Fluor, Ferr Phos, Nat Mur	Loss of elasticity of veins and arteries.
M	Nat Phos, Nat Sulph, Kali Mur, Calc Phos	For rheumatism.
N	Calc Phos, Kali Mur, Kali Phos, Mag Phos	For menstrual pain.
P	Calc Fluor, Calc Phos, Kali Phos, Mag Phos	For poor circulation, chilblains, aching legs, and feet.
Q	Ferr Phos, Kali Mur, Kali Sulph, Nat Mur	For sinus disorders.
R	Calc Fluor, Calc Phos, Ferr Phos, Mag Phos, Silica	For infants' teething pain and to aid dentition.
S	Kali Mur, Nat Phos, Nat Sulph	For stomach upset, digestive and intestinal disorders, and headaches.

Herbal glossary

Term	Definition
Adaptogen	— Balances and restores tone to a particular area
Alterative	— Promotes cleansing and detoxification of blood.
Anodyne	— Herb used to ease or relieve pain.
Anthelmintic	— Used to expel intestinal worms
Antacid	— Helps regulate acid conditions in the stomach.
Antibilious	— Acts on the bile, relieving biliousness.
Antibiotic	— Eradicates viruses and bacteria.
Anticatarrhal	— Eliminates mucus conditions.
Antiemetic	— Stops vomiting.
Antileptic	— Relieves fits.
Antiperiodic	— Arrests morbid periodic movements.
Antipyretic	— Cools system reducing fevers.
Antirheumatic	— Relieves or cures rheumatism.
Antiscorbutic	— Cures or prevents scurvy.
Antiseptic	— Helps prevent putrefaction.
Antispasmodic	— Relieves or prevents spasms.
Antisyphilitic	— Having affect or curing venereal diseases.
Carminative	— Expels gas from the bowels.
Cardiac	— Pertaining to or affecting the heart.
Carthartic	— Cause evacuating from the bowels.
Cephalic	— Remedies used in diseases of the head.
Cholagogue	— Increases the flow of bile.
Condiment	— Improves the flavor of food.
Demulcent	— Soothing, relieves internal inflammation.
Deobstruent	— Removes obstructions.
Depurative	— Purifies the blood.
Detergent	— Cleansing to boils, ulcers and wounds, etc.
Diaphoretic	— Produces and increases perspiration.
Discutient	— Dissolves and heals tumors, abnormal growths.
Diuretic	— Increases the secretion and flow of urine.
Emetic	— Induces vomiting.
Emmenagogue	— Promotes and stimulates menstrual flow.
Emollient	— Softens, soothes inflamed tissue.
Esculent	— Eatable as a food.

Herbal glossary

Term		Definition
Exanthematous	—	Remedy for skin eruptions and diseases.
Expectorant	—	Expulsion of phlegm from mucus membrane.
Febrifuge	—	Abates and reduces fevers.
Galactagogue	—	Promotes secretion of breast milk.
Hemostatic	—	Agent that arrests internal bleeding.
Hepatic	—	For liver diseases, stimulates secretive functions.
Herpatic	—	A remedy for skin diseases of all types.
Laxative	—	Promotes bowel action.
Lithontryptic	—	Dissolves and discharges calculi in urinary organs.
Lymphatic	—	Used to stimulate and cleanse lymphatic system.
Maturating	—	Ripens or brings boils to a head.
Mucilaginous	—	Soothing to all inflammation.
Nauseant	—	Produces vomiting.
Nervine	—	Acts on nervous system, stops nervous excitement.
Nutritive	—	Supplies nutrients, aids building and toning body.
Opthalmicum	—	A remedy for the healing of eye diseases.
Parasiticide	—	Kills and expels parasites from the skin.
Parturient	—	Induces and promotes labor at childbirth.
Pectoral	—	A remedy for chest affections.
Precursor	—	Starts a chain reaction which accelerates growth.
Purgative	—	Causes copious excretions from the bowels.
Refrigerant	—	Cooling.
Resolvent	—	Dissolves boils and tumors.
Rubifacient	—	Increases circulation and produces red skin.
Sedative	—	Nerve tonic, relieves excitement, promotes sleep.
Sialogogue	—	Increases the secretion of saliva.
Stimulant	—	Increases energy, assists functional activity.
Stomachic	—	Strengthens, tones stomach. Relieves indigestion.
Styptic	—	Contracts tissues, blood vessels, arrests bleeding.
Sudorific	—	Produces profuse perspiration.
Tonic	—	A remedy which is invigorating and strengthening.
Vermifuge	—	Destroys and expels worms from the system.
Vulnerary	—	Promotes healing by stimulating cell growth.

**Books are available directly from the publishers.
Send list price plus $2.50 for shipping and handling.**

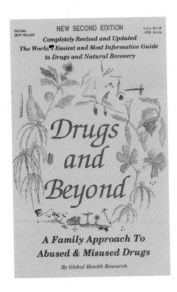

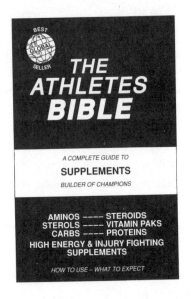

Drugs & Beyond

**A family approach to
abused and misused drugs.
by Global Health Research
$11.95 U.S.A. / $14.95 Cdn.**

An informative and heavily
researched book, construed in
cooperation with some of the top
drug specialists in the world, to
help the general public fully
understand the consequences of
abused and misused drugs. This
book contains illustrations and
clearly designed charts to give
you more information in less
reading time. It covers the full
spectrum of legal and illegal
drugs from caffeine to heroin, the
newest synthetic drugs, and the
latest natural alternatives and
scientific breakthroughs for the
treatments of drug addictions.

The Athlete's Bible

**The proper nutrition to
boost your athletic abilities.
by David Nyholt
$9.95 U.S.A./ $11.95 Cdn.**

If you are an Olympic,
professional, or recreational
athlete, this is the book for you.
Concise, up to date information
on high performance sport
nutrition, aminos, steroids,
sterols, vitamins, carbs, proteins,
high energy, and injury fighting
supplements. Enables you to
boost your athletic abilities,
promote safe muscle tissue
growth, increase strength and
stamina. Enhance energy levels
through proper nutritional
supplementation and reach your
highest possible potential,
without harmful drugs or
chemical additives.

**Books are available directly from the publishers.
Send list price plus $2.50 for shipping and handling.**

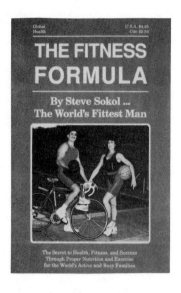

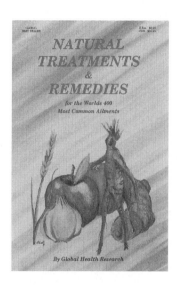

The Fitness Formula
A Must For The World's Active and Busy Families
by Steve Sokol
$4.95 U.S.A./ $5.95 Cdn.

The Secret to Health, Fitness, and Success. Steve Sokol is not only a talented writer and spokesman for numerous health related associations, but also holds over twenty world fitness records. In this book Steve shares with you his proven techniques designed for people of all skill levels, to increase energy levels, mental alertness, health, and fitness. A sensible plan to feel and look your personal best. Building confidence and success through proper nutrition and exercise.

Natural Treatments & Remedies
For over 400 of the worlds most common ailments.
by Global Health Research
$9.95 U.S.A. / $11.95 Cdn.

This informative and heavily researched book is considered to be the most comprehensive and straight forward natural health guide for the worlds most common ailments on the market today. It has been assembled to give you more information in less reading time and to provide the general public with the latest breakthroughs in natural health science at an affordable price. A must for all families that wish to restore health, prevent premature aging, and prolong life, naturally.

**Books are available directly from the publishers.
Send list price plus $2.50 for shipping and handling.**

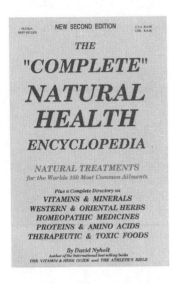

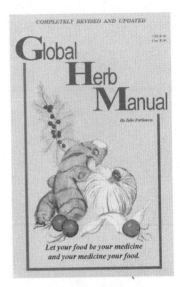

The "Complete" Natural Health Encyclopedia
**A Natural Information Giant
by David Nyholt
$15.95 U.S.A./$19.95 Cdn.**

This concise, comprehensive, and easy to use natural health encyclopedia, is designed to give you more practical information in less reading time. It features the latest breakthroughs in natural health science. Proven and effective natural treatments for over 350 common ailments. 300 western and oriental herbs with their up to date characteristics. 110 Homeopathic remedies. The healing and toxic qualities of 130 foods and spices. Charts on Vitamins, Minerals, Amino Acids, Tissue Salts, and the recommended daily allowances. This book is a must for all people wishing to restore health and prevent premature aging.

Global Herb Manual
**New Sixth Edition
The Latest in Herbal Science
by Zeke Fortisevn
$4.95 U.S.A./$5.95 Cdn.**

This manual is a vast storehouse of knowledge on herbs. Discover the amazing healing and preventative properties of ancient and modern herbs. Plants are mankind's chief method of healing and main source of medicine. This simplified book contains all of the common herbs and characteristics, the effective herbal combinations, extracts, oils and syrups, and their specific functions. Proven herbal cleansing diets, over 50 herbal treatments for the world's most common ailments, plus a comprehensive index and a complete herbal glossary.